The Superbeing Protocol

The Superbeing Protocol

The Step-by-Step Guide to Becoming
Super-Healthy, Super-Fit and
Living an Extraordinary Life

by André Khabbazi

For Jack Colvin

Let me tell you what I think messes up the mind the most: doing less than you can. It causes all types of psychic damage. Being less than you can be, trying less than you can try, somehow damages your mind, your self image.

— Jim Rohn

Table of Contents

Introduction 1

Chapter 1: From Desperation to Destiny 5

Chapter 2: It All Starts With Your Health 15

Chapter 3: The Superbeing 30-day Challenge 35

Chapter 4: Superfoods for Superbeings 55

Chapter 5: How to Make Your Dream Come True 79

Chapter 6: Entering the Zone 97

Chapter 7: Choose Happiness 117

Conclusion 135

Appendix 137

About the Author 153

Introduction

Writing this book is a dream come true for me. It has always been a dream of mine to find a way to help people, to inspire people, to be of service in some way and to empower people to be the best that they can be. I truly believe that we all have greatness within us, if we just allow ourselves to let go of all our fears, doubts, worries and all those limitations that are holding us back from achieving our dreams.

This book is dedicated to anyone who is struggling, tired, worn out, unmotivated, hopeless and hungry to turn his or her life around in a positive way. It is specifically for the person who is sick of living a mediocre existence and fed up with living below their potential. It's time for you to live the life you were born to live. A life filled with abundance, super-health, success, love and joy.

I don't know what your situation is right now. I don't know what you're going through or anything about your circumstances. But I know this: once you make an affirmative decision that you will do whatever it takes to turn your life around, and commit every day to doing the little and conscious things necessary to accomplish your dreams, you will start to see miracles unfold in your life. My own life is proof.

You deserve to be successful. You deserve to be healthy. You deserve to be wealthy. You deserve to be happy. You deserve to be in a loving relationship, live in a beautiful house, drive a beautiful car and have all of your dreams come true!

I created the Superbeing Protocol out of desperation. I was desperate to change my life and tired of living below my potential. I was tired of getting up every day and going to a job that I hated, a job that was making me sick. I was tired of feeling inadequate, tired of being out of shape, tired of being broke, and most of all sick and tired of looking at myself in the mirror and seeing the face of someone who had given up hope.

The Superbeing Protocol is about taking small steps to achieve big dreams. It's about making small adjustments that enhance the quality of your life, your health and your circumstances. It's about taking consistent action towards your goals and improving your life 1%— every day in every way. It's ultimately about reinventing yourself, honoring your commitments and becoming phenomenal in every area of your life.

I believe in you! I believe that you can create whatever it is that you want in life, if you show up, start small, take consistent action and have faith in your vision. Sure, it will take time. It will take effort, consistency, focus and a strong, unwavering belief in yourself to create the kind of life you have always dreamed of living. But it's worth it. You're worth it! Your dreams are worth it!

During our journey together, there will be days when you don't feel like working, when you don't feel like putting in the time, or making the effort or giving your best. There will be days when you will want to give up, quit and surrender. All I ask is that you show up. Just show up. I guarantee you that if you just show up on the days that you don't feel like doing anything, you will transform your life. The results will take time, but you will see them. You will create the life that you have always dreamed of living and gain the confidence necessary to continue despite any obstacles that you will face. *Consistency creates clarity.*

I am so honored and grateful to be on this life-changing journey with you. Nothing will give me more joy than seeing all of your dreams come true. I know how hard it is to change, but I also know that anything is possible when you're committed to creating a better life for yourself.

The lessons and techniques that I will share with you in this book have completely transformed my life, the life of my family and thousands of others who were ready to make profound changes in their life. On this journey of self-discovery I will lead the way, guide you, inspire you and motivate you to keep going when you don't feel like it. I will be the voice whispering in your ear, urging you on to stay consistent, focused and positive.

This is your time to shine. This is your moment to stand up and affirm that you're special, powerful and phenomenal in every way! Let's get started. Best of luck!

down. My body was collapsing. My lungs were bleeding. My liver was dead. I was dying. I had no motivation to do anything. I would work all night and sleep all day. Then repeat the process. Every night the same shit, alcohol, cigarettes, drugs and partying.

I've lived a crazy life. I've always been impulsive, highly emotional and a tad reckless. I've always been attracted to the darker, edgier side of life. I couldn't just smoke 3 cigarettes, I had to smoke 60. I couldn't just drink 2 shots of tequila; I had to drink 10, sometimes 20 in one night. I couldn't just take 1 hit of ecstasy— I had to take 6. There was no in-between with me. It was all or nothing. It's always been that way.

I've learned now that I can get through anything that life throws at me. I've learned that I am in control of my destiny. I'm in charge of my life. I realize that I have a choice every morning when I wake up: I can either take small steps to improve my life or I can fall back into the same bad habits that caused me so much pain in the past. It's your life. You decide how it's going to turn out. Every decision you make from this moment on, will either pull you towards greatness or push you further away from your dreams!

It's Time to Change or Die

If you want different results stop doing the same stupid stuff.

— Eric Thomas

Life can get dark, if you let it. It's easy to slip off the edge if you're not prepared to stand strong, persevere and fight for your life. It sucks to feel stuck. It sucks to be controlled by the pangs of addiction. It sucks to go through life feeling empty and tired and sick. It sucks to be broke. It sucks to be on welfare. It sucks to take a handful of food stamps to the grocery store to buy milk, cheese and crackers for your kids. It sucks to not have a car, to take the bus everywhere you go. It sucks to live in a bad neighborhood. It sucks to be overweight with low self-esteem. It sucks to cry yourself to sleep every night because you can't afford to buy your children food. It sucks to not know your Life Purpose, when you can yet feel deep down in your gut that you have something special to share with the world. I get it! It sucks. I know. I've been there.

I know what it feels like to wake up every morning hung over with my mouth glued shut. I know what it feels like to sleep in a house with roaches crawling on the walls. I know what it feels like to live an empty life, surrounded by bottles and ashtrays. I know what it feels like to look in the mirror and not recognize my reflection. I know what it feels like to not have enough money to feed my family. I know what it feels like to beg for pennies. I know what it feels like to walk the streets at 4am with nowhere to go, drunk, insane, scared and lonely. I've been there. I know what it's like. I'm not trying to over-dramatize my experiences. I just want you to know that there is always a way out of the darkness.

As I indicated in the introduction, I don't know what your circumstances are at this moment, but what I do know is this: You can get out. You can fight your way out. It's going to take time, but it's possible. With commitment, it's probable. You can change your life and live your dreams; it's not too late. Do you hear what I'm saying? I'm telling you not to give up hope. Never lose hope. It's not too late to change your life, and profoundly.

There is always a way out. This isn't just a saying— this is real. Don't surrender. Stay strong. Your life is important! You're important! You're special, beautiful and amazing! The world needs your gifts, your talents, your love, your humor, your charisma, your joy, your laughter and your compassion. The world needs you.

I never believed that I would ever make it out of that bar alive. I never believed that I would ever give up my addictions. I never believed that I was worthy enough to live my passions, share my gifts with the world and accomplish my dreams. I never believed it, until the day I decided to change my habits, create a better life for myself and pursue my destiny.

I made a list of the habits that were causing me the most pain and decided one morning to annihilate them, one at a time.

I quit smoking. This was tough for me. I started small. Baby steps. One cigarette at a time. Here's the formula that worked for me: I kept a journal and wrote down how many cigarettes I smoked every day for one week. Once I saw on paper how many cigarettes I actually smoked every day, I was astonished. If you smoke a pack a day, set a goal for yourself to cut that in half by the end of the week. This is a gradual process. Take small steps, write them down and hold yourself accountable. The process is going to be challenging at first, but stick with it. You can do it!

Another very effective tactic that worked wonders for me was exercise. Whenever I had the urge to smoke, I went on a walk, or a short run, or did 20 pushups. I did something physical. A physical activity that would make me sweat and breathe and feel good about myself. I would go outside in the sunshine, do a few jumping jacks, jump rope or play tennis. I did anything physical to take my mind away from reaching for that cigarette and lighting it up. The results were remarkable! Try this for a week and you will see what an effective method this is. Remember, gradual is good.

I quit drinking alcohol. This was a game-changer for me, and the hardest habit to break. I worked at a bar and made drinks for a living. It was tough at first, but I got through it. I got through it. The first thing I did was eliminate hard alcohol; I only allowed myself to drink wine and beer. This was a gradual process: I couldn't just quit cold turkey, I had to take it slow and methodically work through it. Once again, exercise saved my life, helping me when the craving for alcohol came on strong. I would take long walks, run, stretch, breathe, pray, jump rope, play tennis, swim, sweat, anything I could to stay active. The longer I exercised, the more I would sweat, and the less I wanted to drink.

You already know this intuitively: Exercise will save

your life. Make it a goal to exercise and sweat a little every day, go on a walk around the block or a slow jog, do a few pushups or some light calisthenics. Start small and make gradual adjustments as you go along. The key is to start. That's it! Just show up and do a little bit every day. Everything you do counts! Give it a try and see for yourself how amazing you feel.

I quit my job. This was the scariest thing I've ever had to do in my life, but I had to do it. It was either quit or die! I'm not being dramatic. I'm being honest. I was scared to death. I was scared to leave my job: I had responsibilities, bills, kids to feed, a dog, rent to pay, a wife to support. But this was life or death for me—it had to be done. I had to muster up the courage and do it. That toxic environment was killing me, ruining my relationship with my wife and poisoning my mind. Leaving that bar opened up a whole new world for me. A huge weight was lifted off my shoulders. I started dreaming about my future again, exercising, eating healthy foods and rebuilding my mind, body and spirit. What a staggering difference, just to have made that decision.

The day I left my job was the best day of my life. I was scared, but relieved. Nervous, but excited. I knew intuitively that I had made the right decision. I'm not suggesting that you quit your job, but if you're in a situation that is literally killing you, you must consider it. If your soul is dying, if your heart is telling you that you need to change careers, to get a new job, or start your own business and work for yourself—do it! Do it now, and don't look back. Your life will never be the same again. You will have taken charge!

Action Kills Fear

We all must suffer one of two things, the pain of discipline or the pain of regret.

—*Jim Rohn*

You're special, beautiful, talented and brilliant! This isn't empty flattery. This is the truth and I want you to accept it. I know that you want to change your life and make a difference in the world. I know that you want to help people, share your ideas and leave your mark. I know that you want to be a role model to your friends, family, and every person you come in contact with. I know that your dreams are meaningful to you. I know that you're hungry and ready to commit to accomplishing your goals and highest ideals. I know that you lie in bed at night and dream about your future. The fact that you're reading this book tells me that.

I also know that it's hard. I know that it takes time, intense focus, commitment and the willingness to overcome some extreme obstacles. I know that it's hard to quit self-destructive habits. I know that it's hard to have faith in your abilities and believe in yourself. I know that it's hard to get past your fear and step into your greatness, but you can do it! How? Action.

Action kills fear. Taking consistent action will tame that fear that is bubbling up inside of your stomach. Action can silence that voice that is telling you that you're not good enough, talented enough, good-looking enough, smart enough, thin enough or strong enough. Action will subdue that voice, no matter how loudly it tells you to give up, surrender, move on, quit, stay in bed, sleep, hide, or run away.

Action annihilates fear! It's the little actions you take every day that are going to determine whether you succeed or fail in life. Those small, mundane actions that don't seem important in the moment are going to add up over time and give you the life you always dreamed of living. The micro-actions that go unnoticed by everyone around you, but accumulate over time and turn into something big. A vision. A goal. A dream. A reality.

I'm not talking about taking quantum leaps towards your goals or running a marathon or scaling Mt. Everest on your first trip. I'm talking about taking one small step. An inch, not a mile. I'm talking about showing up and getting started. I'm talking about lacing up your tennis shoes and walking around the block. I'm talking about writing the first sentence of that book you have always dreamed of writing. I'm talking about painting one picture. I'm talking about drinking one glass of fresh vegetable juice. I'm talking about writing down one goal you want to accomplish on a piece of paper. I'm talking about reading one page of an inspiring, uplifting, motivational book.

This is a process—your dreams are not going to happen overnight. It will take time for you to master the mundane and commit to these simple disciplines. However, when they are compounded over time, they'll add up and bring you everything you have ever dreamed of.

CHAPTER 2
It All Starts With Your Health

The food you eat can be either the safest & most powerful form of medicine or the slowest form of poison.

— *Ann Wigmore*

There's nothing more important than your health! I know that you've probably heard this a thousand times before, but it's the truth. It's worth reflecting on at a more-than-superficial level: If you don't have your health, you don't have anything. Just ask anyone who is suffering from any health issues or has battled any type of illness in their life. I'm sure they will tell you that keeping yourself healthy—physically, mentally and spiritually— should be a top priority.

It can be life-transforming to realize that everything you eat, everything you drink and every thought you think will have a profound effect on the quality of your life. If you eat bad food, loaded with refined sugar, saturated fats, preservatives, additives or any other type of chemicals, it's not likely you will have the energy, enthusiasm, or motivation to go after your goals and accomplish your dreams.

If you indulge in alcohol, drink 5 Red Bulls every morning before work, and smoke a pack of cigarettes every afternoon on your lunch break, it's highly unlikely that you will have the motivation, vitality or passion to attack your goals and give your absolute best towards creating the life you have always dreamed of living.

I'm not saying that you should never eat a slice of pizza, or have a hamburger every once in a while, or a beer. No. That's not the sticking point. The key is that you need to become conscious of the little choices you make every day, that have a profound impact on your health and quality of your life. Every choice you make is either pulling you further away from your goals or pushing you towards them. There's no in-between.

The change can be as simple as drinking a glass of water every morning, instead of drinking 3 cups of coffee, or going on a walk, instead of sitting on the coach surfing the Internet or watching TV for 6 hours. Those are the small, consistent adjustments that you can make in your life that will determine whether you're healthy or sick, rich or poor, happy or miserable! I want to emphasize again: small adjustments over time can produce big gains.

I encourage you to remind yourself daily that everything you do matters, everything you do counts, everything you do or don't do will have an effect on your physical, emotional and spiritual health. This is your life we are talking about! It's time to get moving, get healthy, get motivated and take those small steps towards creating a life filled with abundance, vibrant health, wealth and happiness.

I was addicted to alcohol for 14 years, I smoked 2 packs of cigarettes a day, and every night at 4am, I pulled into the McDonalds drive-through and ordered a Big Mac, extra large fries and a Coke. How do you think I felt in the morning?

It's worth answering: I felt terrible! I had no motivation to do anything. I couldn't even get out of bed until 2pm. I've alluded to it earlier, but my situation bears reviewing: I was tired, unmotivated and sick. My body was dying and my mind was falling apart— and there didn't seem to be anything I could do about it. I was caught in a trap. Quicksand. I couldn't see any way out. My body was severely dehydrated. My mind was dark and my soul was dead.

It wasn't until I reached my breaking point (or maybe even a little after) that I decided that I had to do something about my health. I *had* to make changes. I had to figure a way out. I had to make my health the #1 priority in my life or I was going to die. I was suffering. I was depressed, negative, angry and sad. I was poisoning my body, every day with bad food, alcohol, cigarettes, drugs, and negative thoughts. It was a terrible time.

This was the lowest point in my life, but I made it out alive by taking one step at a time, climbing, inch-by-inch out of the darkness. And into the light.

You Were Born to Move

If exercise came in pill form, it would be plastered across the front page, hailed as the blockbuster drug of the century.
— *John J. Ratey*

Exercise saved my life! I was a very active kid and played competitive tennis throughout my childhood. I trained an average of 2 hours every day on the court and supplemented my workout with running, jump roping, weightlifting and calisthenics. Staying active was a huge part of my life growing up, and it still is to this day. At any point in my life when I feel depressed, unmotivated, lethargic, stressed out, sad, angry, or uncertain about my future, I always start exercising to snap me out of it—and it always helps. Guaranteed. I always feel 100% better after I get my heart pumping and get moving and sweating. Exercise is the greatest drug on earth.

Undoubtedly, you already know that exercising on a regular basis makes you feel better. You know intuitively what you need to do to stay healthy, get fit and live a long life, but so many people don't do it. They let themselves go. They stop caring and give up. They become comfortable. They may start exercising, then stop. Then they repeat this process over and over throughout their lives. I know that it's difficult to change certain habits; I've been there and I can sympathize with you. It's tough, but it's possible to change. And those changes deliver life-altering results. I promise.

Look around you and you will see people who have given up hope and settled for a life of mediocrity. People who have lost their passion for living. Lost that spark they once had. Their eyes are dead. They're tired, worn out, sick, solitary and despondent. **Please, don't let this happen to you.** I will show you a better, healthier way to live. Stay with me—let's do this together. I challenge you to push yourself to continually improve your life, by exercising, eating healthy food and thinking positive uplifting thoughts. This isn't some woo-woo dreamer's quest. This is real life.

You have more in you than you realize, and you're capable of achieving so much more than you could ever dream of. If you want to be healthy, successful and live up to your true potential you need to get moving, get active, get fit, get motivated and get excited about your future. Keep that spark alive inside of you and one day it will turn into a flame. Your life will shine with a beautiful light that you would have never dreamed possible.

Exercise will save you! And soon enough, beginning with small efforts, you'll start to crave its benefits, and delight in the feeling exercise gives you. It will change your life in so many positive ways. Here are just a few of the many benefits exercise will have on your life:

1. **Relieves stress.** Exercise is a stress killer! It knocks stress dead in its tracks, by increasing norepinephrine, a chemical that can moderate the brain's response to stress. Any time in my life that I have felt stressed out (to the point of having a panic attack), the first thing I do is go on a walk, or a jog, or a light run. I get active and get moving as quickly as possible, because I knew from experience that if I stayed immobile, the stress would increase and send me over the edge. Exercise

cured all that for me—and it will for you as well. That's a promise!

2. **Makes you happy.** Exercise makes you happy. How do you feel after you go on a walk, jog, or run? My bet is that you feel amazing! Exercise is the ultimate happy pill. You go outside, breathe in the fresh air, walk for 20 minutes, work up a sweat and come home smiling. Why? Because exercising releases happy chemicals into the brain, like dopamine. If we stay active, walk, jog, run, lift, jump, stretch and move, we increase our brains production of dopamine, which stimulates feelings of pleasure and vitality.

3. **Gives you confidence.** It's very difficult to feel good about yourself if you're not happy with the way you look and feel. A negative self-image or low self-esteem will have a huge impact on the quality of your relationships, your career, your goals, your dreams, and the quality of your life. Exercise gives you the confident feeling of being in control, makes you feel attractive, enhances your wellbeing, makes your skin glow, keeps your weight under control, and makes you feel sexy, strong, and attractive. Not bad, eh?

4. **Motivates you.** Exercise gives you the motivation to be better, to do more and to achieve greatness. Confidence in your body gives you a sense of accomplishment and instills in you the assurance and motivation necessary to accomplish your goals. Once you make a decision to turn your life around and commit to exercising, you'll see it's a key factor in

living your life to the fullest and create the life you have always dreamed of living.

5. **Keeps you healthy.** Exercise brings your immune system back into harmony so that it can reduce inflammation and kill off disease. It delivers oxygen and vital nutrients to your tissues and helps your cardiovascular system work more efficiently. Good exercise gives you more energy during the day and helps you sleep better at night. It puts that spark back into your life and gives you the incentive to eat better food, quit destructive habits, drink clean water, breathe fresh air and create a healthy life for you and your loved ones. It sounds miraculous—and it is.

Everything Counts

Successful people are those who understand that the little choices they make matter, and because of that they choose to do things that seem to make no difference at all in the act of doing them, and they do them over and over until the compound effect kicks in. Those little things that will make you successful in life, that will secure your health, your happiness, your fulfillment, your dreams, are simple, subtle, mundane things that nobody will see, nobody will applaud, nobody will even notice.

— Jeff Olson

Thinking about your goals (and what it might take to achieve them) can be daunting. It's scary to step out of your comfort zone and pursue your dreams. It takes courage, discipline, faith and a strong belief in yourself. It takes commitment, persistence, and the desire to create something meaningful, beautiful and extraordinary.

It's much easier to give into your fears than it is to take that first step, or write that first sentence, or take that first picture, or sing that song, or get on stage, or paint that landscape, or start that business you have always dreamed of starting. Fear will kill you. It will keep you down, choke you and suffocate you until you die with your dream still inside of you. Sure it's easy to give in, but at what cost?

Take that first step! Please! Show up. Take one small step today. Right now. Start the process. Motion creates greatness. Action creates dreams. All it takes is your decision to do something. Go on a walk, make a salad for dinner, skip coffee and make a green smoothie, go to the gym and exercise for 15 minutes, write in your journal, meditate for 5 minutes, write down your goals, visualize your future, wake up 20 minutes earlier, pray. Do something, anything. Everything you do counts!

As I alluded to earlier, it's important that you show up, every day, ready to take action. It's up to you whether that action is 5 minutes or 5 hours, but whatever it is, remember everything you do counts. Every drop of sweat, every little bit of effort, every little action that might go unnoticed is propelling you closer and closer to living the life you have always dreamed of living. So get started, get moving and get consistent!

My Exercise Rituals

Your first ritual that you do during the day is the highest leveraged ritual, by far, because it has the effect of setting your mind, and setting the context, for the rest of your day.
— *Hal Elrod*

I usually wake up around 6 or 6:30 in the morning, drink a glass of water, take the kids to school, come back by 7:15 and start walking. I walk for 30 minutes, then jog all the way to the top of the mountain outside of my house and walk back home. The whole process usually takes about an hour to finish.

I get home, make a smoothie or drink some fresh juice and stretch out on a foam roller for about 15 minutes. In the afternoon, it's time to jump rope. I jump for 20 minutes, do some light calisthenics, pushups, sit-ups, and some deep-breathing exercises to calm my mind and keep me focused.

In the evening I usually mix it up between yoga, martial arts or some light weight-training. I try to get in another hour of solid exercise before I call it a night and retire to bed by 10pm with a good, uplifting, motivational book.

As you can see, I am continually active throughout the day, always pushing myself to give my best, show up and work hard. I also make sure to drink plenty of water, fuel my body with healthy food and get plenty of rest.

I understand that this routine is not for everyone. I am just giving you an example of what I do and how dedicated I am to getting in the best shape that I possibly can. Everyone is different. Everyone has different goals and reasons for exercising. For me it was life or death. There was no other way. Exercise saved my life, so I know the positive impact it can have on someone's future. Regular exercise can totally transform your life if you give it a chance and you stay consistent. And it's essential for me to say: it becomes something you look forward to, not look at as a dreary obligation.

How I Got in the Best Shape of My Life in 21 Days

So I skipped a day at the gym. What's a day? Hey, it's just a cheeseburger, what's the fuss? The difference between success and failure is not dramatic. In fact, the difference between success and failure is so subtle, so mundane, that most people miss it.

— Jeff Olson

There's a mountain outside of my house that I stared at every morning when I woke up. I'd hiked to the top a few times, but I'd always wondered what it would feel like to run all the way up to the top without stopping. I've always wanted to conquer that damn mountain, cross the finish line and raise my hands up in victory. I knew that if I could just run up to the top of that mountain every morning, I would get in world-class shape and feel better than I've ever felt in my life.

The stage was set. I woke up one morning, determined to accomplish my goal. I took a deep breath, laced up my shoes, grabbed my water bottle and walked out of the house towards the base of the mountain.

[Days 1-7] Phase 1: Painful

If you want to be good at something you must do it every day. You must work tirelessly towards your goal. You need to wake up every day and make a conscious decision to simply do more. Every step towards achieving your goal, no matter how big or small that step is, is a step in the right direction.
— Robert MacDonald

I was excited to start my journey. I wanted to push myself to get in phenomenal shape, but I knew intuitively that if I had any chance of conquering this mountain and sticking to my new program, I would have to start slow, take small steps, and be consistent. I made a commitment to myself that I was going to show up at the base of the mountain, every morning for the next 21 days, no matter what!

I started walking at first. It was painful. I had to stop every few feet to catch my breath. The altitude kicked my butt. My mind was telling me to quit. My legs were shaking. The top of the mountain seemed so far away, but something inside of me kept pushing me along. One foot in front of the other. I kept moving, until I reached the top. I bent down, rested my hands on my knees and tried to catch my breath. I was exhausted, but I made it. I showed up and I did it. My work was done for the day.

The next 7 days were pretty much the same. I inched along until I reached the top. Some days felt better than others, but I could tell something was changing inside of me. As the days passed I could catch my breath much easier. I wasn't as winded. My legs felt strong and my mind stopped trying to convince me to quit. I was determined more than ever that I was going to run to the top of the mountain without stopping and nothing was going to stop me from achieving my goal.

[Days 8-14] Phase 2: Things Are Looking Up

When life knocks you down, try to land on your back.
Because if you can look up, you can get up. Let your reason
get you back up.

— Les Brown

By day 8 things were looking up! This was becoming a routine for me. I would wake up in the morning, look out my window and stare out at the mountain. I would visualize myself running up to the top, fit, strong, and unstoppable. I knew what I had to do and I did it. I got ready, walked outside and prepared myself for the climb. I started pushing a little harder, picking up the pace. I would jog a few feet, walk, rest and jog again until I reached the top. Once I reached the top I would throw my hands up over my head and clench my fists. Yes! I did it!

As I alluded to earlier, 80% of being successful at anything is showing up. If you can show up, then the rest will take care of itself. It takes courage to show up every day when you don't feel like it, but it's the only way that you're going to create the life of your dreams. You're going to have to show up on the days that you don't feel like working and take a small step. Remember, it's the little things you do every day, compounded over time, that will determine where you will end up in life.

I showed up every morning ready to attack the mountain. I was starting to see little changes in my body. I lost a few pounds, my muscles were tightening, my lungs expanding. I could breathe deeply and recover much faster than when I first started. I started feeling superhuman, my mind was becoming clear, focused and charged with positivity. I was overwhelmed with a deep sense of gratitude every time I reached the top. I also loved being outdoors and immersed in nature. I felt connected to a higher power and for the first time in my life I actually felt like I could accomplish anything!

When I made it to day 14, I was jogging halfway up the mountain. I would jog the first half, then walk the rest of the way up. My body was sore, but I didn't let that stop me. I knew that if I truly wanted to get in the best shape of my life then I was going to have to move past my comfort zone and push myself to a place that was unfamiliar. A place where I could grow, a sacred place, beyond limitations, doubt and fear.

Conquering this mountain was becoming a spiritual experience for me, a time to reflect, imagine and dream. What's your mountain? What's it going to take for you to get up, get moving, get inspired and make your dreams come true? This is your time, don't let it slip. Show up and make it happen!

[Days 15-21] Phase 3: It's a Miracle

Here's what I discovered: The minute you turn this cycle around and start motivating yourself, you'll see immediate rewards. Maybe not monetary ones, not yet. But it's how you feel about yourself that's of the greatest value. Discover all you can do. See how much you can earn, how much you can share, how much you can start, how much you can finish, how far you can reach, and how far you can extend your influence.

— Jim Rohn

By the time I made it past the second week (without missing a day), it was smooth sailing! By day 18, I could jog all the way up to the top of the mountain without stopping. I couldn't believe it. It seemed so far off in the beginning. When I finally made it to the top, I raised my hands in victory, wiped the tears from my eyes and screamed with joy. I had accomplished something big! I did it! I stuck to my plan. Showed up every day. Inched along and made it to the top without stopping. A private victory.

I honored my commitment to myself and also figured out the formula for success, something concrete that I could carry with me throughout my life; show up, take small steps, stay consistent, be patient, have faith and believe that you can accomplish anything you set your mind to. It's a miracle!

Step Into Your Greatness

The Two Choices We Face

Each of us has two distinct choices to make about what we will do with our lives. The first choice we can make is to be less than we have the capacity to be. To earn less. To have less. To read less and think less. To try less and discipline ourselves less. These are the choices that lead to an empty life. These are the choices that, once made, lead to a life of constant apprehension instead of a life of wondrous anticipation.

And the second choice? To do it all! To become all that we can possibly be. To read every book that we possibly can. To earn as much as we possibly can. To give and share as much as we possibly can. To strive and produce and accomplish as much as we possibly can. All of us have that choice.

— Jim Rohn

I want you to understand in the deepest part of yourself, that you have greatness within you. Maybe you haven't had the chance to express it, but it's inside of you—greatness is ready to come out. It *wants* to come out. Your talents, your gifts, your love, your passion, your enthusiasm, your discipline and your greatness want to come out. It's time for you to take charge of your life, get that spark back and regain your passion for living.

I want you to be fit, strong and happy. I want your life to overflow with success, abundance and vibrant health. You deserve that. Time is moving so fast. If you're going to make a change in your life, do it now while there's still time. It's not too late, I promise. Dig deep within yourself, step out of your comfort zone, and aggressively attack your goals, every day with the tenacity of a lion.

It doesn't matter how old you are, or how young, or how thin, or how overweight, or how much money you have, or if your father was in your life, or if you grew up poor. It doesn't matter. The past is gone. Finished. All you have is now. Today. This moment to either shine or hide. What's it going to be? I want you to excel, to grind it out and show the world that you have what it takes to create miracles, that you have comeback power, that you're special, amazing and phenomenal in every way.

You have so much potential. What are you doing with it? Why are you wasting it? You have the potential to soar, to fly and to create the most beautiful life imaginable for yourself and for your family. I want you to start demanding more from yourself, every second, every minute, every day. Your dreams are at risk. Your health is at risk. Your life is at risk.

Now let's get to work on your dreams. Let's create a plan and commit to showing up every day, no matter what! Remember, 80% of being successful is showing up—even when you don't feel like it. Let's really do it this time. No more excuses. I want you to get excited. I want you to get hungry and find that passion that will catapult you to success in every area of your life!

CHAPTER 3
The Superbeing 30-day Challenge

There are only two ways to live your life. One is as though nothing is a miracle. The other is as though everything is a miracle.

— *Albert Einstein*

Congratulations on making it this far! I want you to know that going into the first 10 days of this program that it will be challenging at times. You may feel some resistance, you might feel tired, sore and sluggish. There will be days that you will want to quit, give in, surrender and go back to your old ways of living.

Be on guard. Stay out of your head, which can often whisper negative thoughts and fears. Instead, follow your heart and think about your dreams. Remind yourself every day that you deserve to be successful in every way. Pain is temporary. Fight through the initial pain and a whole new world will open up for you. Stick with me, believe in yourself, and you're going to experience a sense of joy that you have never felt before.

For the next 30 days I want you to think about your life. What is it that you truly want? Think about it, see it, visualize it. I want you to be healthy, strong and powerful. I want you to radiate vibrant health, feel amazing and get in the best shape of your life. Surely you want this too. You can do it! You're ready. Let's get started.

[Days 1-10] Walking, Water, and Juicing

I have always been delighted at the prospect of a new day, a fresh try, one more start, with perhaps a bit of magic waiting somewhere behind the morning.

— *J.B Priestley*

I love to walk! Walking will change your life. I walk every day for at least 30 minutes. I love to get up in the morning, drink a glass of water or some fresh green juice, get dressed, grab my iPod and hit the trails. There's something special about being outside, early in the morning, breathing in the fresh air, feeling the warm sun on my skin and walking through the mountains. Pure bliss!

Step 1: Start Walking

I would love for you to start walking, every day. It doesn't matter how far you walk. You can walk down the street and come right back if you want. The point is to get started, get moving and get active. For the next 10 days I want you to walk for a minimum of 5 minutes every morning. I want you to plan this out and see it through, no matter what comes up. I want you to get ready the night before, and have everything you need to make this experience successful for yourself. Have everything laid out and ready to go: Your shoes, socks, sweat pants, shirt, water bottle, headphones and whatever else you need to get started. This is your plan of attack. No excuses. Have everything ready in the morning, walk out the door and start walking.

Remember, this is not a marathon or a race. All I'm asking you to do is show up and put in your 5 minutes a day for the next 10 days. No more, no less. If you can do this and not skip a day, then you are well on your way to achieving greatness. Dig deep within yourself, get excited, motivated and pumped up to improve your life. Your dreams are within reach. Push yourself, commit to walking every day for the next 10 days and don't settle for anything less. Don't give in to your fears, fight the temptation to fall back into your same routine. If you want your life to change, you have to change something. You have to do something different today than you did yesterday. Start walking!

Step 2: Drink Plenty of Water

The first thing I do when I wake up in the morning is drink a full glass of alkaline or spring water. Drinking a minimum of 8 glasses of water daily is probably one of the best things you can do for your health. Water will help flush out the toxins that have built up in your body, giving you more energy to exercise. It will also help keep your immune system strong, relieve fatigue, and keep you happy, healthy and hydrated. There's a wonderful book that I would recommend titled You're Not Sick, You're Thirsty by F. Batmanghelidj. This is a life-changing book on the health benefits of drinking water.

Once you make it a habit of drinking a sufficient amount of clean, pure water every day, you will see results, immediately. Your skin will glow, you will have more energy, you will sleep better, your headaches will go away, you will be less constipated, more alert and have more motivation to go on your daily walk.

For the next 10 days, I encourage you to wake up in the morning and drink a full glass of water before you go on your walk. Water first. You can keep a water bottle next to your bed, so when you wake up you can enjoy it immediately. This habit alone has the potential to change your life, improve your health and keep you focused on all of the positive things in your life.

I know that it's not always easy to jump out of bed in the morning and grab a glass of water, especially if you're used to drinking coffee, or a soda or some other caffeinated beverage. I'm not asking you to give up those things. All that I'm asking you to do is to make sure that you drink enough water throughout the day to keep your health in balance and your body functioning properly.

Also, if you can, try to drink water that has been filtered in some way. You want to always drink clean, pure water. If possible, try to stay away from tap water. Tap water contains a lot of chemicals that may be harmful to your health. I personally love alkaline water, or spring water. If you're on the run, then it's fine to grab a bottle of water, but try to avoid plastic containers if you can—there are a myriad of chemicals in plastic that you don't want to be drinking.

Remember, if you're thirsty, then you're in the beginning phase of dehydration. I know it sounds simple to drink a glass of water, but it's one of those things that's easy do and also easy not to do. If you want to keep your body, mind and spirit working in harmony then drink a minimum of 8 glasses of water every day for the next 10 days. Your body will thank you!

Step 3: Juice It Up

Nothing is better than drinking a glass of fresh fruit or vegetable juice early in the morning, after you have finished with your walk. Most of us just don't get enough nutrients, vitamins, and enzymes in our diet to keep us performing at a peak level. If you are going to go after your dreams, you need to be at your best, physically, mentally and spiritually. I want you to—and you will want to—have energy, stamina, focus and the clarity to attack your goals.

So for the next 10 days, please add one glass of organic, green juice to your diet. Try juicing a cucumber with 1 stalk of celery and a handful of kale. If you have a hard time drinking fresh green juice then it's perfectly fine to have a piece of fruit thrown into the mix for flavor. This may sound like a lot for you, but it's actually not that difficult once you get started. At the end of this book I have listed some of my favorite juice and smoothie recipes for you to try. Not only do they taste amazing, but they are incredible for your health and will keep you performing at your best.

In January 2010, I fasted on green and fruit juice for 30 days. It was one of the most incredible experiences of my life. After the first couple days my food cravings went away and I was overwhelmed with a sense of euphoria. I'm not suggesting that you juice-fast right now, but that might be something that you look into down the road if you are serious about getting into the best shape of your life.

For now, I just want you to drink one glass of fresh green juice, every day for the next 10 days, on top of what you normally eat and drink. Don't make any drastic changes to your diet. I want you to start slow and stay consistent. If you have a juicer, that's great! You can use that, or buy juice at your local grocery store. Just make sure that it's always pure and fresh, no additives. Fresh juice for the next 10 days.

What's so amazing about juicing is that you will see the benefits right away. Research suggests that juicing helps strengthen the immune system, facilitates weight loss, increases energy levels, makes your skin glow and keeps your bones strong. It will also keep you sharp, focused and clear as you move one step closer towards accomplishing your goals. You'll be amazed—and delighted!

[Days 11-20] From Good to Great

It only takes one extra pushup, it only takes one extra mile, it only takes one extra effort, one extra something to get from where you are to where you want to be.

— Eric Thomas

Take a moment and give yourself a hug or a pat on the back for making it this far. I'm serious. You have done what 95% of the population refuses to do or ignores, which is take the first step towards creating the life of your dreams. Congratulations! You're amazing and don't ever forget that.

This is the time when things get interesting. The halfway point, between good and great. This is where you might encounter a lot of resistance, fear, anger and sadness. Be on guard. Protect your dream. Stay on course. Stay active and never give up. Remember, pain is temporary. I can't emphasize this enough—*Pain is temporary!* You will get through this and your life will never be the same again. I promise you! Hang in there and stay positive. You can do it!

Step 1: Give Extra Effort

Develop the habit of applying consistent extra effort, vision and focus in everything you do. Once it becomes a habit, it will be second nature. Imagine if your attitude, your focus, your engagement with other people and your perseverance were all just a little better. Ask yourself what that would be worth.

—Quinton McCauley

Hopefully you've been walking, drinking water and have added some fresh, organic juice into your life. If you have, that's awesome! If not, don't beat yourself up, go back to Day 1 and get started. There's still time to start your journey. Make it happen for yourself. Keep that vision of excellence at the forefront of your mind and never give up on your dreams. Remember, take action and stay consistent. One step at a time until you reach the top.

I feel like you're ready to take the jump, make the leap and commit to taking your life to the next level. Going from good to great is all about giving a little extra effort. Pushing yourself a little bit further. Demanding a little bit more. If you're walking every morning for 5 minutes, I would love if you could extend the time to maybe 15 or 20 minutes.

This is the time that I need you—and you need you—to stay strong, focused and determined. This is your time to shine—don't get complacent and forfeit the gains you're already making. Activate your discipline. You have so much inside of you. Your discipline will save your life. Give a little push, increase the amount of time you're exercising by 5 or 10 minutes every day. Stay with the water and the juice and keep a positive attitude.

Maybe think about some other exercise options as well, something that would take you out of your comfort zone, but that you can discover that you love. Activities like yoga, Pilates, kickboxing, swimming, cycling or tennis. The amazing thing about these activities is that they don't feel like exercise. You have a chance to get ultra-fit, burn calories, lose weight, build muscle and have loads of fun doing something you can enjoy and love. That's the secret! Get fit doing something you love.

It doesn't require that much more effort to move from being good at something to being great at something. It only requires a little more effort than what you've already been giving. Just a little extra. If you made a commitment to yourself to do 20 pushups every day, then bump it up to 30 or 40. Don't go overboard with this and burn yourself out. Remember what I said earlier: take small, consistent steps in the direction of your dreams and never give up until you reach your goals.

If you like to run a mile every afternoon after work, then make it a mile and half and see how you feel. I'm talking about making a 1% improvement in your life, pushing yourself just a little bit more, giving a little extra oomph, every second, every minute and every day.

It takes guts to get out of bed every morning, drink a glass of water, lace up your shoes and start walking. It takes courage, discipline and a strong work ethic to show up every day and put in work. It's not easy. If it was easy, everybody would be healthy, wealthy and happy.

Step 2: Record Your Life

Always carry a notebook. And I mean always. The short-term memory only retains information for three minutes; unless it is committed to paper you can lose an idea forever.

— Will Self

I can't tell you enough how excited I am that you're taking the steps, every day to creating the life of your dreams. You're getting up, drinking water, exercising, drinking juice, pushing yourself to be the best that you can be. Think about how amazing that is! Think about how far you've already come. Congratulations! I'm so ecstatic that you're taking control of your life, creating your future, showing up every day and giving your best. You're awesome!

Now would be a good time to get a journal so that you can record your thoughts, experiences and feelings. If you already have one (and write in it every day), then you're already on track. Good for you! But if not, consider getting a journal or a notebook and start writing in it for 5 minutes every day. It doesn't have to be long, just a paragraph or two will be fine. Write down your thoughts, get them out of your head and down on paper.

Writing is therapeutic. It will help relieve stress, keep your mind sharp, focused and clear. It's also a good way to record your goals and dreams. Writing your goals down on paper and seeing them in your own handwriting has a powerful effect on your subconscious mind. I will go more in-depth into goal-setting techniques in a later chapter, and clarify the best ways to write down your goals.

Journaling is also a good way to write down all of the things that you're grateful for in your life. It's so easy to get stressed out, worry, get negative, depressed and down on yourself. It's so easy to forget that life is precious, beautiful and amazing. There are so many things in your life that I'm sure you're grateful for—writing them down can remind you of the richness of your life.

Write them down in your journal, the little things: your health, your family, your home, the fact that you have food to eat, clothes to wear, your mind, your happiness, the beautiful blue sky, fresh air, your friends and your parents. Write them down on paper. Take 5 minutes and make a list. Don't worry about spelling or punctuation.

Just write, breathe and smile. I will go deeper into the power of gratitude in a later chapter, but for now just find a few minutes every day to record your thoughts in your journal.

Step 3: The Reading Miracle

Miss a meal if you have to, but don't miss a book.

— *Jim Rohn*

Reading is a game-changer. It changed my life! I didn't realize it then, but the day I started reading was the day I started to transform my life. The day I walked into Barnes & Noble and picked up a copy of Think and Grow Rich by Napoleon Hill was the day that I started climbing out of the darkness and into the light.

From that moment I was hooked on reading. I made a life-altering decision to read a minimum of 15 minutes every night of an inspiring, uplifting, educational book. This habit alone changed the course of my life, inspired me to pursue my passions and gave me the courage to go after my dreams.

Reading 15 minutes every day will give you the extra motivation you need to stay on track and continue in the direction of your Life Purpose. All it takes is the right book to change the direction of your life, reignite your passion, motivate you and empower you to go after your dreams. Start reading. Take 5 minutes out of your day and focus on reading a book that inspires you, empowers you and uplifts your spirit.

It's important that you read every day! Like everything else we have discussed so far, it's better to read 5 to 10 minutes every day, than it is to read a novel in 3 hours and never read again. Staying consistent, persistent, and dedicated is the key to success in every area of your life. Once you master this philosophy, there will be no limit to what you can accomplish. Start reading. Expand your mind, knowledge and curiosity. Read great books that empower you, inspire you and uplift your spirit.

I have listed a few of my favorite life-changing books in the Appendix section of this book. These are the books that have had the most impact on transforming my life. I hope that you get a chance to read through some of them and make reading a top priority in your life. Best of luck!

[Days 21-30] From Great to Phenomenal

I'm not the smartest. But you will not out work me! I wake up every morning at 3 o'clock!

— *Cal Ripken*

My life turned around the day I realized that I was responsible for the way my life had turned out. I created it. I created it with my thoughts, my actions, my behavior, my laziness, my attitude and my excuses. I was responsible for everything.

Once I came to this realization and stopped blaming my circumstances, my mother, my father, my boss, my kids, my wife, the government, my past and everyone else in the world, my life turned around. I stopped making excuses and started making better choices.

I started exercising every day, meditating, eating better food, stopped drinking alcohol, stopped smoking, stopped blaming, stopped making excuses, quit my soul-sucking job, moved out of the city, started writing down my goals and started taking massive amounts of action towards my destiny.

Your life is in your hands. You already know intuitively what you need to do to become successful. These next 10 days are about taking the limits off what you think you can accomplish, and pushing yourself to be the best that you can be. There are no limits!

Step 1: Get Ultra-fit

Can you imagine what I would do if I could do all I can?
— Sun Tzu

It's time to get ultra-fit! Don't let this scare you. You're ready to make the jump. You've put in the work, taken the small steps, pushed past the pain and made a commitment to improving your life in every way. I want you to take your fitness from great to phenomenal! I want you to feel your best, look your best and create the best life imaginable for yourself. Your transformation is already on its way—a new world awaits.

What would your life look like if you gave 120% every day to getting in the best shape of your life? What would that feel like? It's time for you to leave a legacy. To be an inspiration. A role model. To leave your mark. You've waited long enough. It's time for you to start taking massive amounts of action in the pursuit of your dreams.

If you want to take your life to the next level, then I want you to start thinking about ways to get in world-class shape. I want you to start thinking about making your exercise routine your top priority. I want to challenge you to get out of bed a half-hour earlier than you normally would and make a decision to put in some serious roadwork.

This is a different mindset! I'm talking about stepping out of an "average" mentality and stepping into your potential, your greatness, and your genius, so that you can fly, soar and create miracles in your life.

Every day that you wake up healthy is a miracle. You have been given another chance to create your future, chisel away at your fears and become the best that you possibly can. Think about that as you move through your day. You've been given another chance to create something meaningful for yourself. Don't settle for anything less than your best!

Step 2: Thinking Your Way to Success

With every thought we think we either summon or block a miracle.

— Marianne Williamson

I'm a firm believer in the power of positive thinking. I can tell you from my own experience that positive thinking works miracles if you give it a chance. I spent 14 years working in a nightclub in Los Angeles and the only way I made it out of that dungeon alive was by filling my mind with positive, uplifting thoughts.

It wasn't easy. There were nights when my mind was dark and I felt like giving up, running away and hiding. There were many nights when I felt like I was never going to escape the trap that I was caught in, but through those hard times I always reminded myself to stay positive, have faith and believe that things would change.

It's not easy to stay positive when you're struggling, angry, sad and you resent the world. It's not easy to pretend things are fine when you know deep down that your life is a mess. It's a challenge to stay positive during hard times. I know it's difficult, but it's necessary. You need to dig deep within yourself and try to keep a positive outlook on your life.

Nothing is set in stone. Things will change in your life if you have the right attitude, but if you let negativity consume your mind then you're setting yourself up for failure. You're creating your own misery, digging your own grave and preventing yourself from achieving greatness.

I want you to start watching your thoughts as they slip through your mind. I want you to spy on yourself for the next few days, without judgment. Just see what comes up. What are you thinking about? What consumes you? Are a majority of your thoughts positive or negative? How do you feel? If you are in good spirits, then there's a good chance you're thinking positive, uplifting thoughts. That's a good gauge—your emotions will give you a clue about what is happening inside of your mind.

Any time a negative thought creeps up on you, it needs to be cancelled immediately, before it can take root and grow into something bigger. The remedy can be as simple as saying "CANCEL" or "STOP" and replacing it with a positive, uplifting thought or affirmation. I will talk more about the power of affirmations in a later chapter and clarify any misconceptions you might have about positive thinking, visualization, affirmations and the power to use your mind to create the life of your dreams.

Cynthia K. Chandler, counseling psychologist at Indiana State University and Cheryl A. Kolander, assistant professor at the Department of Health at the University of Louisville in Kentucky, have some amazing observations which appeared in Education Digest, January 1989:

"Beliefs or thoughts held in the mind on a conscious or subconscious level cause the body to respond physiologically or behaviorally. Positive self-communication provides a key to effecting a healthy lifestyle ... Students often say negative things about themselves, diminishing positive mental energy. A thought that is in the mind is to some degree believed and can eventually manifest itself in behavior.

"Thought stopping is an effective response to self-defeating thoughts and emotions. Each time a negative thought comes to mind, students can immediately say to themselves "stop." This command acts as a distractor and interrupts the flow of self-defeating thinking. It is a simple command that will help break a persistent habit. Thought stopping can interrupt any type of unpleasant thought. It can aid in breaking obsessive or fearful thoughts such as thoughts of failure, inadequacy, panic or anxiety, painful memories, or recurring impulses such as nail-biting or over overeating.

"Thought stopping can be followed by thought substitutions of positively reassuring or self-accepting statements. Each negative thought the student stops can be followed by a positive one. For example, "I'm so stupid" can be stopped and replaced with "I am smart, and I can do it"; or "I'm a fool" can be replaced with "I learned something, and I am wiser because of it." Substitute "I don't have what it takes" with "I have the courage to give it my best shot.""

Don't underestimate the power of your thoughts. Your thoughts create your world. Your thoughts have the power to turn your life completely around. Positive thinking works! It worked for me and has worked for thousands of other people throughout history. Remember, your thoughts create your reality. If you make the effort to change your inner world, then your outer world will change.

Step 3: Meditation

The mind can go in a thousand directions, but on this

beautiful path, I walk in peace. With each step, the wind blows. With each step, a flower blooms.
— *Thich Nhat Hanh*

I once heard a guru say that by meditating just 5 minutes every day, you could completely change the course of your destiny. I believe it! Meditation is so powerful; it brings a sense of stillness, peace and calm to your life. It gives you unshakable confidence, enhances your mood, and boosts your immune system.

I don't want to complicate things too much by insisting that you sit cross-legged for 2 hours every morning on a rock and chant Hindu mantras before the sun rises. No, that's not what I'm talking about. I simply want you to find a quiet time for yourself, free from distractions. A time when you can be alone with your thoughts, relax your mind and connect to your higher self. Simple!

You can use this quiet time to meditate, pray, write in your journal, visualize or just sit quietly and breathe—it's up to you. There's no wrong or right way. You can do whatever you want. It's your time. All I ask is that you do it for a minimum of 5 minutes every day, for the next 10 days and stay consistent with it. After 10 days you can decide for yourself if you want to continue the process, but at least give it a chance and see if it works for you.

I prefer to meditate first thing in the morning, before life gets hectic, stressful and chaotic. I usually sit in a chair, relax my body, close my eyes and do about 5 or 10 minutes of deep-breathing exercises. I always feel better after I meditate—the effects are instantaneous. I feel centered, calm, ready and excited to tackle my morning.

It's one thing to talk about meditation, or try to explain it, but meditation is really something that needs to be experienced. You need to do it, go through it and feel it to truly understand the benefits. It's a lot like experiencing the feeling of love; you don't really understand it until you go through it.

We spend a majority of our life worrying, stressed-out, preoccupied with the future, on the move and in a constant state of panic. We owe it to ourselves to take a moment to breathe, slow down, calm our nerves, relax and be in the moment. Once you experience the magic of meditation, you will be hooked for life.

In a study published last year, scientists at the University of California in Los Angeles and Nobel prizewinner Elizabeth Blackburn found that 12 minutes of daily meditation for eight weeks increased telomerase activity by 43 percent, suggesting an improvement in stress-induced aging. Blackburn, of the University of California, San Francisco, shared the Nobel Prize in medicine in 2009 with Carol Greider and Jack Szostak for research on the telomerase "immortality enzyme," which slows the cellular aging process.

Remember, your health is the most important thing you have, you owe it to yourself to take a few minutes every day to slow down, breathe and rejuvenate your mind, body and spirit!

CHAPTER 4
Superfoods for Superbeings

Superfoods are both food and medicine; they have elements of both. They are a class of the most potent, super-concentrated, and nutrient-rich foods on the planet; they have more bang for your buck than our usual foods. Extremely tasty and satisfying, superfoods have the ability to tremendously increase the vital force and energy of one's body, and are the optimum choice for improving overall health, boosting the immune system, elevating serotonin production, enhancing sexuality, and cleansing and alkalizing the body. Superfoods meet and exceed all our protein requirements, our vitamin and mineral requirements, glyconutrient (essential polysaccharide sugar) requirements, essential fatty acid requirements, immune system requirements, and so much more. Nourishing us at the deepest level possible, they are the true fuel of today's "superhero." Superfoods make having The Best Day Ever fast, easy, fresh, and fun!

— David Wolfe

Superfoods are a special category of the most powerful, healing foods on the planet. They are low in calories, packed with nutrients, and are loaded with antioxidants, enzymes and essential nutrients that your body needs to function at its best. They come in every shape and size:

- Fruits and Nuts
- Greens
- Bee Products
- Seaweed
- Herbs

Superfoods are for anyone who wants to feel amazing, have boundless energy, detox, lose weight and get in the best shape of their life. They're for anyone who would like to nourish their brain, bones, muscles, skin, lungs, liver, heart, kidneys and immune system. This is what superfood expert, David Wolfe has to say about the benefits of adding superfoods into your daily diet:

"When you bring superfoods into your body, your energy changes, and as a result your focus of attention will shift as well. It is likely that you will reassess your values (what you consider important). You may see the world with more energy behind your eyes: with the added boost, it becomes easier to live in a state of appreciation. Over time, you will likely perceive the world as a more amazing place than ever before, because you will feel better more often. I eat super foods every day, and they make me feel the best ever, always!"

I've learned that it's nearly impossible to get

depressed when you eat healthy, drink enough water, exercise and supplement your diet with superfoods. Try blending some kale, raspberries, goji berries and coconut water together into a green smoothie, drink it and tell me how you feel.

If that's not enough to make you feel incredible, try adding a little cacao powder, a pinch of bee pollen and some maca powder into the mix and blend them all together into a super smoothie.

I can tell you from my own experience that once I started adding superfoods into my diet, my life took on a whole new meaning. I had more energy, better focus, and an intense desire to stay that way. I never realized that I could eat food that had the capability to heal my mind, body and soul. Incredible! Once you start adding superfoods into your diet, you will see positive results immediately.

You've heard it before: "You are what you eat." Everything that you put into your mouth is going to affect how you feel. Too many people in this world are living with poor health, low energy, low self-esteem and chronic pain.

Obesity is on the rise among adults and children in the United States. A recent study published in the American Journal of Preventive Medicine this month predicts that 42 percent of Americans will be obese by 2030, and 11 percent of the population will be severely obese, or roughly 100 pounds overweight by that year.

Approximately one-third of the U.S. adult population and 17 percent of American adolescents are obese.

It's up to you to change your destiny. You have the power to create the life of your dreams, enjoy vibrant health and live pain-free, by incorporating superfoods, exercise, positive thinking and all of the other suggestions I have made throughout this book into your daily life!

I'm going to share with you some of my favorite superfoods and super herbs that I absolutely love and incorporate into my diet every day. I usually blend them together into a smoothie, tea, or eat them raw. All of these ways will work. I have listed some superfood smoothie and tea recipes for you at the end of this book and hope that you take the time to look through each one and try them out for yourself. Not only are they incredible for your health, but they taste amazing!

André Khabbazi

Turmeric Is King

Could there really be one herb that does it all? One herb that simultaneously works as an antioxidant, modulates inflammation, supports joint health, detoxifies the body, protects the cardiovascular system, promotes normal cell growth, supports mental clarity, regulates the bowels, balances stress hormones, supports healthy blood sugar metabolism, promotes wound healing, and even boosts serotonin production?

An incredible body of growing research suggests that yes, there is such an herb! It's Turmeric!

— Taryn Forrelli

If I had only one choice of one superfood, or herb, or spice that benefits me the most and keeps me healthy throughout my life, it would be turmeric! Turmeric is king! In my opinion there's nothing better for keeping your body healthy, flexible and strong.

Turmeric is a miracle spice that gives curry its yellowish color. It has been used in Ayurvedic medicine throughout India as a medicinal herb for thousands of years to treat a myriad of ailments. Curcumin is the main active ingredient in turmeric; it's a powerful anti-inflammatory and has incredible antioxidant properties.

One of the most comprehensive summaries of turmeric was published by the respected ethnobotanist James A. Duke, Ph.D., in the October, 2007 issue of *Alternative & Complementary Therapies,* and summarized in the July 2008 issue of the *American Botanical Council* publication *HerbClip*.

Reviewing some 700 studies, Duke concluded that turmeric appears to outperform many pharmaceuticals in its effects against several chronic, debilitating diseases, and does so with virtually no adverse side effects. Here are just a few of the diseases that turmeric has been found to help or alleviate:

- **Alzheimer's disease:** Duke found more than 50 studies on turmeric's effects in addressing Alzheimer's disease. The reports indicate that extracts of turmeric contain a number of natural agents that block the formation of beta-amyloid, the substance responsible for the plaques that slowly obstruct cerebral function in Alzheimer's disease.

- **Arthritis:** Turmeric contains more than two dozen anti-inflammatory compounds, including six different COX-2-inhibitors (the COX-2 enzyme promotes pain, swelling, and inflammation; inhibitors selectively block that enzyme). By itself, writes Duke, curcumin—the component in turmeric most often cited for its healthful effects—is a multifaceted anti-inflammatory agent, and studies of the efficacy of curcumin have demonstrated positive changes in arthritic symptoms.

- **Cancer:** Duke found more than 200 citations regarding turmeric and cancer and more than 700 for curcumin and cancer. He noted that in the handbook *Phytochemicals: Mechanisms of Action,* curcumin and/or turmeric were effective in animal models in prevention and/or treatment of colon cancer, mammary cancer, prostate cancer, liver cancer in rats, esophageal cancer, and oral cancer. Duke said that the effectiveness of the herb against these cancers compared favorably with that reported for pharmaceuticals.

How can you get more turmeric into your diet?

You can purchase turmeric capsules at your local health food store, or get the powder in the spice section of your local supermarket. Turmeric is very cheap and it tastes great! I sprinkle turmeric powder on pretty much everything that I eat: rice, pasta, salads, avocado, beans, and more. I also add a pinch of turmeric into every smoothie that I make, or juice the root in the winter with ginger and use it as a cold buster.

Bee Superfoods

Bee products are an amazing class of superfood that can complement our health for the rest of our lives.

— David Wolfe

Bee products are considered the healthiest foods on the planet. I've been using bee products for the past 10 years and highly recommend consuming bee products on a daily basis. Bee superfoods taste great and are inexpensive!

The main thing to keep in mind when purchasing all of your bee products is to make sure that everything you buy is raw, wild and organic. You don't want your honey, bee pollen, propolis, or royal jelly filled with additives, pesticides or chemicals!

Let's start with my favorite:

Bee Pollen — Bee pollen is considered to be one of the most complete foods found in nature. It contains nearly all of the nutrients required by humans to survive: at least 22 amino acids, 18 vitamins, 25 minerals, 59 trace elements, 14 fatty acids, 11 carbohydrates and 11 enzymes. It's a rich source of protein (approximately 40% protein) and is loaded with B vitamins, as well C, D, and E.

Bee pollen also contains an abundance of minerals: Calcium, Phosphorous, Potassium, Iron, Copper, Zinc, Sodium, Sulfur, Magnesium, Manganese, Silica, and Titanium.

Honeybee pollen is the richest source of vitamins found in Nature in a single food. Even if bee pollen had none of its other vital ingredients, its content of rutin alone would justify taking at least a teaspoon daily, if for no other reason than strengthening the capillaries. Pollen is extremely rich in rutin and may have the highest content of any source, plus it provides a high content of the nuclei's RNA [ribonucleic acid] and DNA [deoxyribonucleic acid].

— Institute of Apiculture, Taranov, Russia

You can purchase raw, organic bee pollen in the refrigerated section of your local health food store. It's inexpensive and it tastes amazing! You can eat a teaspoon in the morning for breakfast, or add it to your power smoothies for lunch. Give it try!

Raw Honey — Organic/wild raw honey is nature's true energy booster. It's loaded with antioxidants, minerals, and enzymes and is one of the most healing foods on the planet. Honey is also a powerful immune-system booster and has natural antibacterial properties to help fight off disease, heal cuts, colds, sore throats, coughs, ulcers, burns and wounds.

Dr. Peter Molan, professor of biochemistry at Waikato University, New Zealand, has been at the forefront of honey research for 20 years, and has this to say about the healing benefits of honey:

"The remarkable ability of honey to reduce inflammation and mop up free radicals should halt the progress of skin damage like it does in burns, as well as protecting from infection setting in. At present, people are turning to honey when nothing else works. But there are very good grounds for using honey as a therapeutic agent of first choice."

I personally love honey. I eat raw, organic, unfiltered

honey every day. I take a spoonful in the morning and use it as a natural sweetener throughout the day. As you already know, honey tastes amazing! It's incredible for your health, and should be something that you consider adding into your diet.

Propolis — Propolis is a remarkable healer. Bees gather propolis from the leaf buds of trees and certain vegetables to disinfect the beehive and seal cracks. Propolis is a natural antibiotic and prevents infection, protecting the immune system from free-radical damage. It is a rich source of amino acids, minerals, vitamin C and vitamin B.

Propolis has been used throughout history to treat a wide variety of ailments, from arthritis to helping fight winter illnesses such as the flu, colds, and various allergies.

Some studies suggest that when applied to infected areas topically, it may be used against bacteria and viruses and other microorganisms. Propolis has antimicrobial action on both gram-positive and gram-negative microorganisms. It contains constituents that increase membrane permeability and inhibit bacterial motility. It is commonly used for wound infection and other illnesses.

Propolis is a true healer and one of the most powerful natural shields on earth against viruses. It can be taken in many different ways: capsules, lozenges, pure alcoholic extract, spray, syrups, or mixed in with raw, organic honey.
— Excerpt from NaturalNews.com's article, "Bee Propolis: Nature's Healing Balm With Immune Boosting Properties" by Katherine East

I enjoy taking it in the morning, mixed with bee pollen and raw honey. It tastes great and will give you enough energy, strength, stamina and focus to last throughout your whole day!

Royal Jelly — Royal Jelly is probably the least understood superfood, and one of the most potent. Some believe that Royal Jelly is "the fountain of youth and beauty." It's loaded with B vitamins and is a rich source of protein (50% protein), carbohydrates (20% carbohydrates), and fat (14% fat). Royal Jelly is reserved exclusively for the Queen bee to eat. It has been used throughout history to restore vitality, rejuvenate the body, and promote a long life. Consider the following:

The greater nutritional significance of Royal Jelly is the fact that the anatomical and functional differentiation of the female larvae is totally dependent upon the nature of their diet in their early development stage. In the larvae stage, they are absolutely identical and feed on Royal Jelly for the first three days after hatching. The fertilized eggs give rise to females, which are either sexually immature small worker bees or large, fertile Queens. From the fourth day on, only the special larvae selected to become the Queen continues to be fed with Royal Jelly throughout her entire life, while the worker bees are fed on regular honey and pollen. The fascinating discovery by apiculturists was that nutrition was the only distinctive difference between the worker bees and the Queen. The Queen bee is a mother of a quarter of a million bees, and amazingly lays over 2,000 eggs in a single day, a total more than twice her own body weight. The life span of the Queen lasts 4 to 5 years, contrary to the considerably shorter life of the workers, an average of 3 months or less.

Taking your daily dose of Royal Jelly will keep you young, healthy and fit throughout your life. Consuming less than half a teaspoon daily is a perfect way for you to achieve longevity, and receive a powerful dose of C, E and B vitamins. Royal Jelly is truly a miraculous superfood! I've been taking it regularly for the past 5 years, combined with honey, bee pollen and propolis and would considerate it one of the most powerful, healing foods on the planet.
         — Excerpted from the article "Fresh Royal Jelly" by Y.S. Royal Jelly and Honey Farm.

André Khabbazi

Medicinal Mushrooms
(Reishi & Chaga)

Medicinal mushrooms have super tonic and adaptogenic properties that allow you to consistently (even multiple times daily) ingest their nutrient-medicines that strengthen immunity; help fight allergies, asthma, and cancer; improve core vitality; and confer many other valuable gifts.

— David Wolfe

Reishi — Reishi mushroom, also known as Lingzhi mushroom or the "mushroom of immortality," has been used throughout Asia for its medicinal purposes for over 2,000 years.

In Life Extension Magazine a recent article by Emily Steiner on "How Reishi Combats Aging" had this to say:

"There is now a wealth of impressive data that demonstrates reishi's life-extending properties, but also its significant ability to stimulate brain neurons, search and destroy cancer cells and prevent the development of new fat cells in obese individuals. As an example of the growing science supporting reishi, researchers using laboratory mice have detailed life span extension of 9% to more than 20%, the equivalent of 7 to nearly 16 years in human terms. As if these targeted benefits were not sufficient, reishi's numerous compounds show a therapeutic effect on asthma, allergies, diabetes, autoimmune diseases, Alzheimer's and Parkinson's diseases, liver disease and more."

Scientific research suggests that reishi mushrooms possess anti-tumor, anti-diabetic, anti-parasitic, anti-fungal, anti-inflammatory, anti-viral, anti-allergenic and anti-hypersensitive properties.

Here are just a few of the amazing healing benefits of reishi:

- Boosts the immune system
- May have certain anti-cancer properties
- May help protect and regenerate the liver and fight against chronic hepatitis
- May help calm the mind and help clear depression
- Help delay the aging process
- May help alleviate pain associated with chemotherapy
- Help relieve, cough, asthma and bronchitis
- May help combat cardiovascular disease
- Reduce fatigue

Some experts speak on the many healing benefits of reishi:

Reishi is a supreme immune tonic. Because of its neutral energy, it is fine for anyone to take. It treats immune disorders including AIDS, as it raises the T-cell levels (an index of AIDS and immune disorders). It is also specific for Chronic Fatigue Syndrome. It inhibits bacteria and viruses, treats cancer and tumors and its adaptogenic quality protects the body against stress. It treats heart disease, reduces cholesterol and lowers high blood pressure.

Earl Mindell's Soy Miracle,
by Earl Mindell RPH PHD, page 107

André Khabbazi

In addition to being an effective energizer, reishi is an antioxidant that protects the body from the harmful effects of radiation and free radicals. It contains polysaccharides and other compounds that may combat bacteria and viruses and boost the immune system.

Prescription For Nutritional Healing,
by Phyllis A. Balch CNC and James F. Balch MD, page 469

The third is reishi, currently available in US health food stores. It is said to have been used as a "fountain of youth" elixir for centuries. A novel protein with immunomodulating activity in vivo has been isolated from the mycelial extract of reishi.

Alternative Medicine, *by Burton Goldberg, page 1112*

Reishi is one of the herbs that I cannot live without. I take it every day, and I will continue to take it for the rest of my life. The citations tell you that the benefits of reishi are amazing! I usually purchase reishi powder or a blend of medicinal mushroom powder and make a tea out of it, or add it to my smoothies. Either way, you can't go wrong.

At the end of this chapter I have listed a few of the reputable companies that I order my reishi powder from. These companies have been in business for years and have set the standard for creating quality reishi mushroom powder.

Chaga

Chaga — Also known as the "Gift from God." Chaga has been used by humans for thousands of years to support health. Chaga supports the entire system and it's loaded with vitamin B, flavonoids, phenols, minerals, and enzymes. It promotes longevity and boosts the body's immune system.

Research suggests that it's also a powerful antibacterial, anti-inflammatory, anti-malarial, anti-HIV, anti-cancer, antiviral, anti-fungal and much more.

In his amazing book *Chaga: King of Medicinal Mushrooms,* author David Wolfe states that chaga is rich in antioxidant power and can induce apoptosis, the spontaneous breakdown of cancer cells. It also can "squelch the strong oxidative damage to healthy tissue caused by radioactive chemotherapy."

According to Christopher Hobbs, extracts of chaga were approved as an anti-cancer drug, called Befungin, in Russia as early as 1955 and have been reported successful in treating breast, lung, cervical, and stomach cancers. (Hobbs, 1995)

Mushroom mycologist Paul Stamets writes that, "The betulin concentrations in Inonotus obliguus have shown promise in treating malignant melanoma, completely inhibiting tumors implanted in mice, causing apoptosis of cancerous cells. The extracts are also beneficial as an antiviral, antibacterial and anti-inflammatory. In addition, they are known immune enhancers as well as a liver tonic." (Stamets, 2005)

Here is a list of the many healing benefits of chaga:

- Supports immune function
- May help fight cancer
- Improves mental clarity
- Reduces fatigue
- Helps you sleep better
- Eliminates the effects of stress
- Helps regenerate cells
- May help slow down the aging process
- Helps stabilize blood sugar
- Builds strong blood
- Maintains optimum alkalinity and PH levels
- Improves disease resistance
- Improves digestion
- Manages weight
- Protects DNA
- Improves neurological function
- Suppresses allergies

The easiest way for you to get your daily dose of chaga is either in a capsule or by mixing organic chaga powder in warm water and brewing it as a tea with honey. You can purchase the powder or capsules online or at your local health market. Remember, chaga is a very powerful form of medicine and a truly magical mushroom that has the potential to help heal your body and improve the quality of your life.

Coconut Oil

Coconuts are one of the greatest gifts on this planet. No matter where you are, what you have done, how much you have mistreated your body, fresh young coconut flesh, coconut water, coconut cream, and/or coconut oil can save your life.

— David Wolfe

Virgin organic coconut oil is one of my favorite superfoods. Science is now considering coconut oil a superfood that actually helps the heart by mounting resistance against viruses and bacteria.

Bruce Fife, C.N., and author of *The Coconut Oil Miracle* shares his insight: "Laboratory tests have shown that MCFAs (medium chain fatty acids) found in coconut oil are effective in destroying viruses that cause influenza, measles, herpes, mononucleosis, hepatitis C, and AIDS; bacteria that can cause stomach ulcers, throat infections, pneumonia, sinusitis, urinary tract infections, meningitis, gonorrhea, and toxic shock syndrome; fungi and yeast that lead to ringworm, candida, and thrush; and parasites, that can cause intestinal infections such as giardiasis."

Lauric acid is the most predominant MCT found in coconut oil. Regarding lauric acid, Mary Enig, Ph.D., writes:

"Lauric acid is a medium chain fatty acid, which has the additional beneficial function of being formed into monolaurin in the human or animal body. Monolaurin is the antiviral, antibacterial, and antiprotozoal monoglyceride used by the human or animal to destroy lipid-coated viruses such HIV, herpes, cytomegalovirus, influenza, various pathogenic bacteria, including listeria monocytogenes and helicobacter pylori, and protozoa such as giardia lamblia. Some studies have also shown some antimicrobial effects of the free lauric acid."

The health benefits of coconut oil include:

- Immune system enhancer
- Great at reducing stress
- May help prevent heart disease
- Cholesterol maintenance
- May help with high blood pressure
- May help destroy viruses that cause HIV
- Helps fight off cancer
- Great for your skin
- Amazing for your teeth
- Helps with weight loss
- Relief from kidney problems
- May help problems associated with arthritis
- Natural energy booster
- Lowers cholesterol
- Reduces the risk of Alzheimer's

Coconut oil is one of the healthiest foods on the planet, and it's very inexpensive. You can purchase it in the cooking aisle at the grocery store or in the supplement section or at your local health mart. For the most health benefits, coconut oil should always be purchased either as unrefined, "virgin" or "extra-virgin." I always purchase my coconut oil in bulk from tropicaltraditions.com, in my opinion, they have the best coconut oil on the market.

One of my favorite ways to consume coconut oil is in a cup of warm tea. I also love to mix it in with smoothies, cook with it, rub it on my skin after a shower, use it as a natural deodorant, or just eat a spoonful of it first thing in the morning or at night before bed.

Coconut oil is one of the many superfoods that I consume daily and will continue using for the rest of my life. The healing benefits are incredible—and it's been documented that populations that consume a lot of coconut are among the healthiest people on the planet.

Disclaimer: These statements have not been evaluated by the Food and Drug Administration. These products are not intended to diagnose, treat, cure, or prevent any condition. Always check with a physician before making any dietary changes.

André Khabbazi

Reclaim Your Life

For the past 33 years, I have looked in the mirror every morning and asked myself: If today were the last day of my life, would I want to do what I am about to do today? And whenever the answer has been 'No' for too many days in a row, I know I need to change something.

— Steve Jobs

You have the power to change your destiny, you have the power to get in the best shape of your life, and you have the power to eat healthy, live with vitality and confidence. I've said this before, but its truth bears repeating: you have the power to create the life of your dreams. Start today, and watch the magic unfold in your life, as your dreams manifest into bright beautiful colors.

The day I started adding superfoods into my diet, everything changed for me. I became a different person. I had more energy, I started exercising, eating better, feeling better, and creating better habits for myself. I went from drinking alcohol every night and chain-smoking to drinking fresh green juice, making smoothies and eating food packed with nutrients. The difference is astounding.

What you drink and what you eat affects your life. Please, don't kid yourself into thinking that it doesn't matter. It matters! When I started to change my eating and drinking habits, I started to see the world differently. I started to dream again. Set goals. Meditate. Read. Listen to beautiful music. I was inspired to do more and be the best that I could be. Superfoods changed my life!

That's what I want for you. I want you to take action.

Reclaim your life, starting today. Make a glass of green juice. Eat a teaspoon of coconut oil. Go on a walk. Read a few pages of an inspirational book. Sprinkle a bit of turmeric on your rice. Make a green smoothie. Think positively about your life. Have a spoonful of honey with a pinch of bee pollen. Make a glass of reishi tea. Something. Anything. Just get started! Small steps move to giant leaps.

Here's a list of my favorite superfood websites:

1. **longevitywarehouse.com** — Great place to order any kind of superfood you can imagine. They have an amazing medicinal mushroom blend called "Organic raw mushroom powder blend" and another product that I love called "Immortal Machine Superfood drink mix." Both of these products are amazing!

2. **ultimatesuperfoods.com** — This is a great site. You can purchase organic coconut oil, goji berries, hemp seeds, cacao, seeds, nuts, snacks, Ayurvedic herbs, etc. This place is like the Disneyland of superfoods. Awesome!

3. **davidwolfe.com** — Anything on David's site is worth taking a look at. His raw cacao tastes incredible, and he also offers some of the best books on health, superfoods and nutrition available.

4. **livingnuts.com** — I get all of my raw organic nuts here. Best place on the web!

5. **jingherbs.com** — Great place for all of your Chinese herbs and medicinal mushroom needs.

6. **dragonherbs.com** — Amazing goji berries! The only

goji berries I've ever had that are moist and not dried out. They also sell a product that I highly recommend called "Tonic Alchemy: The Ultimate Supertonic Superfood Blend." Great to add to smoothies or just mix in water for a super shake on the go.

7. **healthforce.com** — The best green superfood powder mix on the market.

8. **warriorfood.com** — Amazing, raw organic protein powder.

9. **liveonlabs.com** — Lypo-Spheric Vitamin C. In my opinion, this is the best vitamin C you can get anywhere.

CHAPTER 5
How to Make Your Dreams Come True

Here's what I've discovered: The minute you turn this cycle around and start motivating yourself, you'll see immediate rewards. Maybe not monetary ones, not yet. But it's how you feel about yourself that's of the greatest value. Discover all you can do. See how much you can earn, how much you can share, how much you can start, how much you can finish, how far you can reach, and how far you can extend your influence.

— Jim Rohn

Dreams do come true for millions of people. Whatever your dream is, just know that it's possible. You can accomplish anything you want in life. My life is testimony. There's a formula for achieving greatness, and once you understand it and follow it faithfully, then anything is possible.

When I was 17, I had this crazy dream of becoming a soap opera star in Hollywood. I wanted to move to Los Angeles from my hometown of Sacramento and I wanted to be a lead actor on the hit TV show *The Young and the Restless*. I had never acted before, but for some crazy reason I wanted to move to Hollywood and pursue a career as a professional actor. I wanted to go to the Emmy awards, walk the red carpet and become a film and TV star. Crazy I know, but that was my dream.

I held that vision in my mind every day. I imagined myself living in LA, auditioning for the show and getting the part. I could feel it so intensely that tears would run down my cheeks. I imagined myself driving on to the lot at CBS, walking through the security line and acting on the show. I imagined this every day for a year.

I wrote down what I wanted on a piece of paper and carried it around with me everywhere I went. It was a crazy dream, but it was my dream—and that's all that mattered. I was going to make it happen no matter what obstacles got in my way. Nothing was going to stop me from landing a lead role on that show.

During that year, I was faced with many challenges and obstacles. I had a kid, got married, worked two jobs and tried my best to support my family. It was a tough time; my wife and I struggled financially, but did our best to keep the family unit together. There were many nights when we didn't have much food or money and had to improvise to make things work, but we got through it.

No matter how dark things got, I always kept my vision. I never lost sight of my goal to become a lead actor on *The Young and the Restless*. A year later I was living in Los

Angeles and made that dream a reality. I was signed to a 3-year deal on the number-one daytime drama in the world and launched my career as a professional actor.

I spent 15 years working as a professional actor in Hollywood. It wasn't always easy. I was hired, fired and out of work for years, but I kept pushing on and did some good work on television, stage and in the movies. I kept improving my craft, studied with the best teachers and stayed persistent. Always keeping my vision protected.

I'm going to share with you a very specific protocol that I learned years ago from an acting teacher of mine, who taught me how to specifically break down film scripts and audition pieces. It's the exact same protocol I use for mapping out my goals and attacking my dreams. It's simple, efficient and in my opinion, the best way to achieve everything you want in life. Let's get started.

What Do You Really Want?

You have the ability to choose which way you want to go.
You have to believe great things are going to happen in your
life. Do everything you can—prepare, pray and achieve—to
make it happen.

— Benjamin Carson

This is the first question that I want you to ask yourself. What do you want? What do you truly want? Until you can answer this question, it will be difficult for you to make any progress in the direction of your dreams. I know sometimes it's hard to answer a question like this. You might feel stuck or unsure about what it is you truly want in life, but I feel like the answer is always there: you just have to quiet your mind and listen to your heart.

I've learned over the years that your intuition is always trying to lead you in the right direction, guide you and help you manifest your greatness. Allow yourself to be courageous, step out of your fear and accept what your heart is trying to tell you.

Your imagination will be your guide. If you're having trouble finding your passion or what it is you want or dream about, spend a few minutes every day just letting your imagination take you on a journey. Find a comfortable, quiet place to sit, close your eyes, take a deep breath and start to visualize your ideal life. What do you see? What moves you? What is your imagination trying to show you?

Sit with it, let it affect your whole being. I've said it before, but I'm going to say it again: you are powerful—

you can create the life of your dreams. Believe in yourself. Get focused, get specific, take action, have faith and never give up. It's time to reclaim your life, take charge and create miracles!

Once you're specific about what it is you want, I want you to write it down on a piece of paper and look at it 3 times a day. This will unleash the power of your subconscious mind and send you flying in the direction of your dreams at warp speed.

Write It Down, Make It Happen

By recording your dreams and goals on paper, you set in motion the process of becoming the person you most want to be.

— *Mark Victor Hansen*

This is so important. It's important to write things down on paper instead of just carrying around your dreams in your head. It's good to have something to look at every day. It will help you stay on track, focused and keep your mind from jumping around from one goal to the next. Write your goals down every day, study them, revise them and ingrain them in your heart.

In the book, *What They Don't Teach You at Harvard Business School,* Mark McCormack tells of a study conducted on students in the 1979 Harvard MBA program. In that year, the students were asked, "Have you set clear, written goals for your future and made plans to accomplish them?" Only 3 percent of the graduates had written goals and plans; 13 percent had goals, but they were not in writing; and 84 percent had no specific goals at all.

Ten years later, the members of the class were interviewed again, and the findings, while somewhat predictable, were nonetheless astonishing. The 13 percent of the class who had goals were earning, on average, twice as much as the 84 percent who had no goals at all. And what about the 3 percent who had clear, written goals? They were earning, on average, ten times as much as the other 97 percent put together.

When I was younger, I was always resistant to writing down my goals. I never really thought that it mattered. I thought that if I had them in my mind, then that would be enough to get me through. It's not enough to just think about your dreams—you need to write them down, be specific about what it is you want and map it out on paper. Create a visual plan for yourself and stick to it, no matter what. Sure you can make adjustments along the way, but stay focused on your goals and see them through to completion.

Find the time to write down your goals every day, study them, and visualize the details of your ideal life, even if it's for a couple minutes. Stay consistent. Resist the temptation to quit after a week or 10 days. Do it every day until you reach your goal, stay motivated, be willing to pay the price for success, and persevere!

The Most Important Question Is "WHY"

If you can't believe in miracles, then believe in yourself.
When you want something bad enough, let that drive push
you to make it happen. Sometimes you'll run into brick walls
that are put there to test you. Find a way around them and
stay focused on your dream. Where there's a will, there's a
way.

— Isabel Lopez

Once you have figured out what you want, and you have written it down on paper, the next step will be to find an emotional reason: the "why" of your want. What's your reason for going after your dream? Why do you want it? What's pushing you, motivating you, and urging you on? There's a reason why you want what you want. What's your reason?

Your emotional reason is going to propel you into taking the necessary action to make your dream become a reality. Take a moment and think about your dream. Who are you doing it for? Be honest with yourself.

There's a reason why you're making the sacrifices every day to make your dreams come true; there's a reason why you're getting out of bed every morning at 6 am and attacking your goals; there's a reason why you go to the gym when you don't feel like it; there's a reason why you stay up until 3am every night working on your business or writing your book; there's a reason why you won't quit or give up when things get hard. The more connected you are to your reason, your "why," the more emotional that reason is to you, the stronger it will be and so will that push to continue working on the days you don't feel like it.

My son is a world-class athlete. We were talking about his dreams and goals, and he told me that he wanted to become a black-belt Brazilian jiu-jitsu world champion. I asked him why he wanted to do that. He said that it was just something that he always dreamed about and wanted to do. I could see the passion in his eyes and knew deep down that he loved jiu-jitsu, that it was a big part of his life, his passion and his true love. His reason "why" was strong and deeply personal to him. He loved the sport. He loved how jiu-jitsu made him feel, and he wanted to be the best!

That's amazing! It's honorable to want to be the best at whatever it is you want to do. I admire that quality, but there's a big difference between wanting to do something because you love it, and wanting to do it because you have to make a name for yourself, so that you can make enough money to feed your 3 children and pull your family out of poverty. You see the difference? I can tell you right now it's going to be harder to defeat the person who has to win the world championship so that he can help his mother move out of the slums of Brazil than it is to beat the person who just wants to win because he loves the sport.

Your reason "why" will be your anchor. It's the thing that will keep you motivated when you don't feel like working. It will be the reason you'll keep pushing yourself every second, every hour and every day until you reach your goal.

Your reason "why" must move you emotionally. Thinking about it should bring tears to your eyes, or make you want to scream or laugh or stand up and shout. The stronger it is, the more emotion you feel thinking about it, the better. Dig deep within yourself. Find your reason to get up every morning and chase down your dream.

What do you want? Why do you want it? Write it down on a piece of paper. Look at it every day. Say it aloud to yourself. Feel it. Imagine it. See the details. Let it affect your spirit. Keep that piece of paper protected. It's sacred. Your dreams are sacred. Carry that piece of paper around with you, everywhere you go. In your wallet, in your purse, in your pocket, in your heart!

André Khabbazi

Make It Happen

I know that I have the ability to achieve the object of my Definite Purpose in life, therefore, I DEMAND of myself persistent, continuous, action toward its attainment, and I here and now promise to render such action.

— Napoleon Hill

Now that you know what you want and you have an emotional reason "why" you want it, it's time to make it happen. I want to take a moment and congratulate you for making it this far and taking the steps to become the best that you can be, physically, mentally and spiritually.

Why not be the best that you can be? You deserve it. Your life changes the moment you decide that you will do whatever it takes to create an exceptional life for yourself. The moment you decide to take relentless action towards your dreams, follow through on your commitments, and never give up until your goals are realized—that's life-changing, and in the most positive of ways.

I'm going to remind you again: greatness comes in small steps. Whatever it is you do, make sure that you do it every day. Stay consistent, persistent and have faith. When I finally grasped this idea and put it to work, my life completely changed. I started putting in the work, setting goals, writing them down on paper, pushing myself every day to improve just a little bit more than the day before. It's the little things that count!

I started focusing on how I spent my time. I realized that time was the most important thing. There are only so many hours in a day. If you want to be successful, don't waste time. It's easy to let 2 hours slip by, numbly watching TV, surfing the Internet, checking emails, or talking on the phone. You need that time to pursue your dreams; don't waste it on frivolous activities that are not contributing to your excellence.

It's time for you to set the standard for everyone else. It's time for you to take charge of your life and regain your passion for living. It's time for you to take action, get excited about your dreams and create the life you deserve. Action will save you. Action will dig you out of the hole that you're trapped in. Action will save your marriage, get you out of debt, heal your body, create the life you have always dreamed of living and save your spirit.

Action is the only thing that counts. You have a choice: You can either show up every day, put in your work and manifest your greatness, or sit back, wait, make excuses, hide, dwell in your anxiety and accept your fate.

Your life is precious! Get up! Get moving! It doesn't matter what you do, just do something that propels you forward, pushes you closer to your dreams and brightens your spirit. One small step. A little baby-action. Do something different today, different than you did yesterday. Plow through your comfort zone and demand more from yourself.

The Little Things Make All The Difference

Little things, little things, are much more important than big things. Big things hit you in the face with their bigness and obscure the little, more important things that really define a life and provide it with delicacy.

— *Lauren Roedy Vaughn*

The little things matter most. This is the truth. The little things that go unnoticed or seem boring at the time of doing them are actually the things that will take you from mediocrity to greatness. For example:

- Writing down your goals every day
- Visualizing your future success
- Repeating your affirmations
- Reading 5 pages of an inspiring, motivational or educational book
- Going to bed at the same time every night
- Waking up at the same time every morning, no exceptions
- Creating morning rituals
- Exercising every day
- Drinking 8 glasses of water
- Drinking a glass of green juice
- Taking a multi-vitamin every day
- Writing in your journal
- Meditating, prayer, gratitude and love

I mentioned that when I was a kid I loved playing tennis. Tennis was my life. I practiced every day and dreamed about playing professional tennis on center court at Wimbledon. I was the #1 junior tennis champ in California and was headed to Florida for the National Clay Court Tennis Championships. Everything was in order. My conditioning was on point, my serve, forehand, almost everything. The only thing that was lacking was my two-handed backhand. I had no confidence in my backhand and didn't know what to do. I needed to do something drastic and fast: the tournament was only a month away and time was running out.

My coach worked with me for a week, feeding me balls, working with me on my footwork, grip and racquet-head positioning, but nothing worked. I was losing confidence in my abilities and was starting to not want to play at all. I was dreading getting on the court and hated the idea of even going to Florida for the tournament.

One morning I decided to walk to the park and hit against the wall. I hated hitting against the wall, it bored me to death, but I needed to do something to get my backhand solid. I figured I'd give it a try. I went the first day and smacked the ball on the wall for about 20 minutes. I made it back the next day and did it again. Still bored. Still hating every minute of it.

I showed up every day for 3 weeks at the same park, at the same time, at the same wall and banged away at my backhand. When it was time to travel to Florida, my backhand was better than my forehand. Solid. Strong. A weapon! I finished that year 17th in the nation, and although I never made it to the center court at Wimbledon, I did learn many valuable lessons that summer:

1. If you want to be successful at anything, you have to show up

2. It's the little things you do every day that count

3. Take action, stay consistent, persist and have faith

4. Get over your boredom and do it anyway

5. Be willing to accomplish your goal, no matter what it takes

6. Take small steps to achieve big dreams

7. Be patient, believe in yourself and do what needs to be done

Before I end this chapter, I want to share with you the most important piece of writing I have ever read. This quote, by my mentor Jim Rohn, changed my life forever and I know it will have a huge impact on the quality of your life as well. Take his words to heart, study them, look at them every day and ingrain them into your heart.

The Formula for Failure

Failure is not a single, cataclysmic event. We do not fail overnight. Failure is the inevitable result of an accumulation of poor thinking and poor choices. To put it simply, failure is nothing more than a few errors of judgment repeated every day.

Now why would someone make an error in judgment

and then be so foolish as to repeat it every day?

The answer is because he or she does not think that it matters.

On their own, our daily acts do not seem that important. A minor oversight, a poor decision, a wasted hour generally don't result in an instant and measurable impact. More often than not, we escape any immediate consequences of our deeds.

If we have not bothered to read a single book in the past ninety days, this lack of discipline does not seem to have any immediate impact on our lives. And since nothing drastic happened to us after the first ninety days, we repeat this error in judgment for another ninety days, and on and on it goes.

Why?

Because it doesn't seem to matter. And herein lies the great danger. Far worse than not reading the books is not even realizing that it matters! Those who eat too many of the wrong foods are contributing to a future health problem, but the joy of the moment overshadows the consequences of the future. It does not seem to matter.

Those who smoke too much or drink too much go on making these poor choices year after year after year ... because it doesn't seem to matter. But the pain and regret of these errors in judgment have only been delayed for a future time. Consequences are seldom instant; instead, they accumulate until the inevitable day of reckoning finally arrives and the price must be paid for our poor choices— choices that didn't seem to matter.

— Jim Rohn

Take action! Don't wait. You've waited long enough. Today is the only day that counts. Life is waiting for you. Share your gifts with the world. Make a commitment to yourself that you will do whatever it takes from this moment on to make your dreams a reality!

CHAPTER 6
Entering the Zone

The difference between try and triumph is just a little umph!
— Marvin Phillips

You've come so far! I'm so proud of you. Keep going, keep pushing and keep dreaming. I hope I'm not belaboring this, but it's so important to understand that you have to put these ideas that I'm teaching you to work. It's not enough to just read the book and put it on the shelf. This book is meant for you to read, study, and use as a guide to making your dreams come true. It's only through action that the rewards—and they are considerable—will come.

These principles that I am sharing with you work, if you use them. I promise. They worked for me at a time in my life when I was shrouded in darkness, hopeless and ready to give up, and they have worked for thousands of other people who were caught in the struggle.

So I challenge you to put these ideas into action, even if only for a few minutes every day. Remember, action is what's going to take you from where you are to where you want to be. The more action you take the better your chances are of succeeding at whatever it is you have chosen to pursue. You only get one life, one chance to leave your mark and to do something amazing!

Make today the day you start the process and take that one step that's going to propel you forward towards your destiny. You showed up here on earth for a reason. It wasn't to just get up every morning, go to a job you hate for 30 years, come home, eat and go to bed. No! You were put here to do much more than that. You were put on this earth to fulfill your Life Purpose, to do something wonderful, amazing and fulfilling.

I want you to start believing in yourself, in your ability to rise up and change your life. I want you to stop making excuses and start making adjustments. I want you to win, succeed and live every day with passion and enthusiasm. You have what it takes! You've already proven that by starting this process, reading this book and following through with the exercises. Now let's take it a step further: let's add the missing ingredient to your success. I call it Entering the Zone!

André Khabbazi

Visualization

Ordinary people only believe in the possible. Extraordinary people visualize not what is possible or probable, but rather what is impossible. And by visualizing the impossible, they begin to see it as possible.

— Cherie Carter Scott

What is visualization anyway? I'm going to make this very simple for you. Visualization or Creative Visualization is a mental technique that uses the imagination to make dreams come true. It's a way for you to attract anything that you want into your life, by seeing it first in your imagination—in detail—then taking the necessary action to achieve it.

It's a proven, scientific fact that "thought" is energy, especially a focused thought that carries with it a high emotional intensity. When you change your thoughts, or the images that you play over and over in your imagination, you change your life.

Visualization is a powerful technique that has been utilized by many top athletes, artists, celebrities, entrepreneurs, and many other successful individuals throughout history including: Will Smith, Oprah Winfrey, Bill Gates, Tony Robbins, Jim Carey, Einstein, Michael Jordan, Wayne Gretzky, and many more.

For instance, Natan Sharansky, a computer specialist who spent 9 years in prison in the USSR after being accused of spying for the US, used the power of visualization for hours every day while locked down in solitary confinement. He played himself in mental chess, saying: "I might as well use the opportunity to become the world champion!"

Remarkably, a short time after his release in 1996, Sharansky beat world-champion chess player Garry Kasparov.

World-champion golfer, Jack Nicklaus has said: "I never hit a shot, not even in practice, without having a very sharp in-focus picture of it in my head." Even Muhammad Ali, arguably the greatest boxer of all time, used different mental practices to enhance his performance in the ring: affirmation, visualization, mental rehearsal, self-confirmation, and perhaps the most powerful epigram of personal worth ever uttered: "I am the greatest."

Your mind is so powerful! You can literally create anything that you want in life by visualizing it first in detail, believing in that image and taking the steps towards achieving it. Visualization techniques turned my life around. I was a depressed teenaged father living on welfare in Sacramento, and through incorporating visualization techniques into my life I was able to pursue my dream of becoming a lead actor on the hit daytime drama *The Young and the Restless* within a short time.

Your dream is possible. If you can see it clearly in your imagination, then you can achieve it. Most people choose to focus on their past mistakes, failures and heartbreaks. They replay the same old movie in their imagination, over and over until it becomes a habit. They become stuck in the past, despondent, unmotivated and give up. Creative visualization gives you another option, the option to create and imagine your ideal future.

What Should I Visualize?

Visualize what it is you truly want. Your goal. Your dream. Your ideal day. Your ideal life. Your deepest desire. Visualize it. See it in your imagination, clearly. See the details. Focus on what you want, instead of dwelling on the things you don't want. What does your dream feel like? What do you hear? What do you see? What do you smell?

I want you to allow yourself to dream about your future. Take your goal and your emotional reason "why" and visualize what it would feel like to accomplish it. You are the star of your own movie. See yourself accomplishing everything that you've ever wanted in life.

If you live in a shabby studio apartment in a bad part of town, visualize yourself opening the door to your new 3-bedroom house in Beverly Hills. If you ride a bike to work every morning and dream about one day buying a Lexus, see it in your imagination. See yourself on the car lot, sitting in your new car. Can you smell the leather? How does your hand feel on the steering wheel? What do you see around you? What time of day is it? What do the keys look like? See the details of your vision. The clearer you can see the details, the faster you will accomplish your dream.

Focus on your dreams and goals and let your past failures fade into the background. Remember, you are the star, the director and producer of your own movie. You make the decisions, you decide what images you replay in your mind every day. This is no fluffy exaggeration: Your imagination is the most powerful force in the universe. You can create anything you want, if you truly believe that you can. See it, believe it, then do it!

3 Simple Ways to Ease Your Way into a Visualization Practice

I'm going to share with you 3 easy ways to get started imagining your ideal life. The most important thing to remember when starting anything new is to show up, take baby steps and be patient with yourself. If you can do those three things, then good things will happen. It's always good to remind yourself that this whole journey that you're on is a process, it will take time, so be patient and keep working at it.

Step 1: Get Started

I like to visualize first thing in the morning, when it's quiet and there are less distractions. It's also a good way to make sure that it gets done. If you wait until the end of the night, there are no guarantees that you will even get around to doing it.

You can start by finding a quiet place to sit, either in a chair or on a cushion. Sit up straight, take a few deep breaths to relax, think about your goals, close your eyes and start imagining your dreams. See yourself accomplishing all of the things that you want in life. See yourself traveling to Paris, walking out onto the deck of your new beach house in Carmel, spending time with loved ones, any of the hopes that really matter to you.

There's no wrong or right way to do this. Some people prefer doing this exercise lying down, while listening to classical music. It really doesn't matter how you do it. The point is to just get started and do it. It's an amazing way to start your morning and leaves you feeling happy, motivated and inspired as you move throughout the rest of your day.

I recommend you start to slowly incorporate this new habit into your life. Start by visualizing for 1 minute, every day for the next 10 days. After that you can increase the time, slowly as you see fit. If it feels good to you, keep doing it. If you absolutely hate it, then stop. There's no need to force the process. Visualization is a very powerful technique and will require some discipline on your part to sit through it, but I can tell you from experience that it works.

Step 2: Write Down the Details

This is a technique that I've utilized over the years to keep my mind focused during my visualization time. Writing down what you want to visualize keeps your mind from jumping around from one image to the next.

When I made the transition from a teenage boy living in Sacramento to a soap opera star living in Hollywood, I used this technique for 15 minutes every day. I found a quiet place to sit, wrote out my plan, took a deep breath, closed my eyes and started imagining myself taking the steps to move to Los Angeles.

I would start by writing down 3 specific images I wanted to focus on that day. Whenever my mind would jump to another image, I would reel it back in and focus on the images that I wrote down. It was a little difficult at first, but after a few days it became natural and a lot easier to stay focused.

Like I said, it's important for you to understand that you have to take this slowly. Start with 1 minute, every day. When you can sit comfortably and visualize what you want for 1 minute, then gradually increase the time you spend imagining your ideal life.

It's all in the details. Try to be as specific as possible when imagining the things that you want. Use all five of your senses. What do you see? Try to see the tiny little details. If you are imagining yourself sitting inside of a blue Lamborghini, then see (and write down) the different colors of the interior. What does the beige leather smell like? What does the engine sound like when you start it up? How do you feel sitting in it? Details!

This will fire up your imagination and send you flying in the direction of your dreams faster than you can ever imagine. Your ability to focus is essential. Write down what you want to visualize and stick to it. One minute every day for the next 10 days.

Step 3: Create a Vision Journal

This is where things get fun! I love the process of creating a Vision Journal. This is very simple, cheap and fun to do. You've already gone through the process of writing down on paper all of the things that you want. You've spent time visualizing yourself achieving all the wonderful things in life that you deserve.

Now you get to take it a step further and find pictures

of the things you want, like a new house, more money, a new car, etc. Tear them out of a magazine or wherever you can find them and glue them into your journal. Sound fun? I hope so.

You can also create a Vision Board that you hang on your wall and look at every day. It's the same idea. I just prefer a Vision Journal, so I can take it with me and look at it everywhere I go. The journal gives me something tangible to focus on and look at every day, to keep me inspired and motivated to keep dreaming.

This is a fun activity you can do with your friends, or your significant other or with your kids. You can make an energizing day out of it. Get a bunch of magazines, a pair of scissors, some glue and get to work. Cut out pictures of the things you want and glue them into your journal. Make this process fun and enjoyable, and most importantly make a habit of referring to your Dream Journal every day so that you can visually see all of the things you want and keep your dreams in focus.

What's cool about having a Dream Journal is that you can constantly add to it. You can carry it with you, write in it, look at it, study it and visualize all the things that you want. It's a fun way to keep your goals and dreams in constant focus, and it works! That's the crazy part about it. It works! Give it a try and see for yourself, you won't be disappointed. Good luck!

Some Final Thoughts on Visualization

See things as you would have them be instead of as they are.

— Robert Collier

Visualization is a powerful tool to help turbocharge your way to success. Most people spend their time worrying, focusing on past failures, traumas, and visualizing the negative aspects of their childhoods. This creates, anxiety, frustration and prevents you from living the life you were born to live.

All of the visualization techniques that I have shared with you in this chapter work, if you use them. Nothing can take the place of action. If you want to become successful and live the kind of life that you deserve, it's important to understand that taking action is the only way that you can make your dreams a reality.

You have to do the exercises, take the steps, and keep pushing forward. Do something different today than you did yesterday. Make one small adjustment in the direction of your dreams. Find a quiet place to sit and visualize your ideal life, even if for 30 seconds or a minute.

Do it every day, and don't stop until you have what you want and become the kind of person that you can be proud of. If you can see it, then you can make it happen. Have faith in your abilities, your imagination, and your vision.

André Khabbazi

The Power of Affirmations

As long as you know what it is you desire, then by simply affirming that it is yours—firmly and positively, with no ifs, buts, or maybes—over and over again, from the minute you arise in the morning until the time you go to sleep at night, and as many times during the day as your work or activities permit, you will be drawn to those people, places, and events that will bring your desires to you.

— Scott Reed

An affirmation is basically a positive statement or declaration that describes a desired situation or what you want to achieve. For example:

"I am the greatest!" This was affirmed daily by the legendary, heavyweight boxing champion of the world, Muhammad Ali. He repeated these powerful words so often, until they were impressed upon his subconscious and he became the greatest!

Affirmations have the ability to rewire our brains by raising the level of feel-good hormones in our bodies, by strengthening our will, by helping us believe in our potential to manifest our goals and dreams. They empower us to take action and play a vital role in breaking the habit of negative thinking.

Write Your Own Affirmations

There's nothing more powerful than writing your own affirmations. For years I would repeat affirmations that I read in books, or online, or picked up somewhere from an article, and that worked temporarily to help me change my negative beliefs about myself. But it wasn't until I started creating my own affirmations that my life really started to turn around and change for the better.

I must admit—at first I was a little intimidated to write down my first affirmation. I had convinced myself that it didn't matter, that it wasn't important, that it was silly, that there was no valid reason why I should create my own affirmations when I could get them from another source.

The day I wrote down my first affirmation was a turning point in my life. Now I write new affirmations in my journal every day. I usually will spend 5 to 15 minutes every morning repeating my affirmations out loud and repeat them multiple times throughout the day until they become automatic.

André Khabbazi

3 Life-Changing Affirmations Techniques

I've made this incredibly easy for you to get started creating life-changing affirmations for yourself. Do not be intimidated by this process: it's simple, easy, fun and very effective!

Step: 1 What Do You Really Want?

The simplest and easiest way to start writing your affirmations is to write a series of "I am" statements that describe exactly what you want to have, feel, or accomplish.

Here are a few examples:

"I am healthy"
"I am happy"
"I am successful"
"I am rich"

It's so important for you to keep your affirmations positive, always focusing on the things you want in your life as opposed to focusing on the things that you're trying to avoid.

For example, rather than writing, "I am not going to smoke cigarettes for the rest of my life," a better choice would be to say, "I am healthy in every way possible" and "I am free from smoking cigarettes" and "I am filled with joy, abundance, and great health."

Keep your affirmations positive and feel free to write affirmations about anything you want: your health, finances, career goals, relationships, spirituality—the things that matter. Your affirmations are for you. They are meant to help you stay positive, change your mindset and help you achieve everything that you want in your life.

Step: 2 Turn Up the Heat

It's very important to be specific when you are creating dynamic affirmations for yourself, so that the universe knows exactly what it is you want to have manifest in your life.

For example, you might create an affirmation like: "I am comfortably and easily earning enough money every month to support my family's financial needs." This is by no means a bad affirmation; it's positive and uplifting, but it needs to be tweaked just a bit to make it even more powerful.

Something more specific, like: "I am comfortably and effortlessly earning 5,000 dollars of extra income every month," will help send a powerful message to your subconscious mind, and quickly send you off in the direction of your goal. Be specific!

I personally love using action verbs ending in "ing" when creating my personal affirmations. Using strong verbs that end in "ing" will automatically bring you into the present moment, by creating a sense of motion, and movement in your affirmation.

Here's a simple example of what I'm speaking about:

"I enjoy spending time with my family." Not a bad affirmation, but let's turn it up a notch and make it more active by using a strong verb, ending with "ing." "I am enjoying spending time with my wife and children."

The latter is much stronger! It brings you into the "now" and gives you a sense that whatever is happening, is in motion. That it's actually happening right now in this moment. This is an amazing technique for amping up your affirmations, and creating dynamic declarations for yourself that actually produce results in your life.

Start now! I challenge you to write out a few affirmations for yourself and see what it feels like. It's empowering, fun and exciting. Don't worry about getting it wrong or messing things up; that's impossible. The more you practice writing affirmations for yourself the easier it will be.

Remember, have fun! This is not a life-or-death situation. This is you sitting down for a couple minutes, with a pen and a piece of paper and spontaneously writing down a few things you would like to have, enjoy, and feel. Have fun!

Step: 3 Affirmations with a Hint of Gratitude

What if your dreams did come true? What would that be like? What would that feel like? Close your eyes for a moment and imagine that all of your goals, everything you ever dreamed of having or doing was real. You accomplished every goal you set for yourself; now open your eyes and write your affirmation from that place inside of you that is grateful for everything that you have been given.

"I am so grateful to be celebrating my 20th wedding anniversary with my beautiful wife and kids."

I want you to celebrate, and cultivate a sense of gratitude in your life for things that you will have in the future. This technique is so powerful, so incredibly amazing that it will transform your life.

Before you write out your affirmations, close your eyes, take a deep breath, visualize what you want, and say "thank you" three times quietly to yourself and start writing.

Just imagine what your life would be like if you repeated "thank you" all day to yourself, while focusing on your goals, writing down your affirmations, and visualizing your future. Your life would be filled with joy, love and abundance in every way.

I will talk more about the power of gratitude in the next chapter, but for now try adding a hint of gratitude to every affirmation that you write.

André Khabbazi

The Formula for Success

Like the formula for failure, the formula for success is easy to follow:

A few disciplines practiced every day.

Now here is an interesting question worth pondering: How can we change the errors in the formula for failure into the disciplines required in the formula for success?

The answer is by making the future an important part of our current philosophy.

Both success and failure involve future consequences, namely the inevitable rewards or unavoidable regrets resulting from past activities. If this is true, why don't more people take time to ponder the future?

The answer is simple: They are so caught up in the current moment that it doesn't seem to matter. The problems and the rewards of today are so absorbing to some human beings that they never pause long enough to think about tomorrow.

But what if we did develop a new discipline to take just a few minutes every day to look a little further down the road? We would then be able to foresee the impending consequences of our current conduct. Armed with the valuable information, we would be able to take the action necessary to change our errors into new success-oriented disciplines.

In other words, by disciplining ourselves to see the future in advance, we would be able to change our thinking, amend our errors and develop new habits to replace the old.

One of the exciting things about the formula for success is that the results are almost immediate. As we voluntarily change daily errors into daily disciplines, we experience positive results in a very short period of time.

When we change our diet, our health improves noticeably in just a few weeks. When we start exercising we feel a new vitality almost immediately. When we begin reading, we experience a growing awareness and a new level of self-confidence. Whatever new discipline we begin to practice daily will produce exciting results that will drive us to become even better at developing new disciplines.

— Jim Rohn

CHAPTER 7
Choose Happiness

Promise yourself to be so strong that nothing can disturb your peace of mind. To talk health, happiness, and prosperity to every person you meet. To make all your friends feel that there is something in them. To look at the sunny side of everything and make your optimism come true.

To think only the best, to work only for the best. To be just as enthusiastic about the success of others as you are about your own. To forget the mistakes of the past and press on to the greater achievements of the future. To wear a cheerful countenance at all times and give every living creature you meet a smile.

To give so much time to the improvement of yourself that you have no time to criticize others. To be too large for worry, too noble for anger, too strong for fear, and too happy to permit the presence of trouble. To think well of

yourself and to proclaim this fact to the world, not in loud words but great deeds.
To live in faith that the whole world is on your side so long as you're true to the best that is in you.

— *Christian D. Larson*

Happiness is a choice. You can choose to be happy at any moment, by making a decision to do things every day that bring you joy. What is it that you enjoy doing? Make a list of all the activities that you love doing. Write them down on a piece of paper, pick one thing from your list and do it every day. For example:

- Exercise
- Eat a healthy meal
- Paint a picture
- Write in your journal
- Watch a funny movie
- Sing
- Spend time with family
- Spend more time in nature
- Meditate
- Help others
- Smile more often
- Read great books
- Practice gratitude
- Go dancing
- Cooking

Life is short! Do what you enjoy. Do what makes you happy and brings a smile to your face. Do it every day. It's often the simple things that we take for granted that bring us the most joy. Go on a walk in nature. Spend time with your family. Take a few moments in the evening to enjoy a beautiful sunset. Pick one thing from your list and do it every day. Choose to be happy!

10 Ways to Live a Happier Life

I am determined to be cheerful and happy in whatever situation I may find myself. For I have learned that the greater part of our misery or unhappiness is determined not by our circumstance but by our disposition.

— Martha Washington

1. **Do Work That You Love.** This is big! We spend most of our adult life working, paying bills, and trying to survive financially. It's so important that you find a way to do work that you enjoy and that makes you happy. Something that you look forward to doing. Something that motivates you, challenges you and makes you grow. I can tell you from experience that it sucks going to a job you hate every day for years and years. Find a way to do work that you love. It's possible. I did it. I quit my job and now I am doing what I have always dreamed of doing. Don't get comfortable in a job that you hate. You have one life to live! Do what you love. Find out what that is and do it now!

2. **Spend Time With Your Family.** It's so easy to get caught up in your work, goals and dreams and forget to spend quality time with your family. Be sure to make time every day for the people in your life that you love, and never take them for granted. Share your love with them; tell your wife, your kids, your mother, your father, your friends and everyone else in your life that you love them. Never withhold your love! Let it

pour out of you, every day. Call your mother and tell her you miss her. Look into your wife's eyes and tell her how special she is. You have this opportunity to show the people you care about how special they are to you. Today is the day. Show them how much you love them!

3. **Relax.** Find time to relax. We are always on the go! It's so important for you to find time during the day to relax a bit, unwind, breathe and calm your nerves. It can be as simple as taking 10 deep breaths, or taking a casual stroll through the park on your lunch break. You can listen to some classical music before bed or meditate for 5 minutes in the morning. I just want you to find a few minutes every day to relax your mind, body and spirit. You can start by taking a few deep breathes every morning before jumping out of bed and starting your day!

4. **Always Give Your Best.** You only have one shot at life. Give your best in every situation. Don't get comfortable. Be proactive and find ways to challenge yourself every day. Give everything you have in you to give and never hold back on your genius. If you want to live a happy, healthy life, then always give your best. Never settle for mediocrity. Always push yourself to give just a little bit more, share just a little bit more and love just a little bit more than you think you can. Doing this will bring so much joy to your life and give you the unshakable confidence to live the life of your dreams.

5. **Exercise.** You should know by now how fanatical I

am about exercising. Exercising is a game-changer. I challenge you to find at least 5 minutes out of your busy schedule to exercise every day. Find activities that you love. You can jump rope, walk, do yoga, play tennis, rock climb, go to an aerobics class, swim, wrestle, play basketball, take a martial-arts class, cycle, do Pilates, run, play golf—there are so many fun activities you can try that don't even feel like exercise. Pick one. Try it out for a week. See if you like it. Sweat. Laugh. Smile and change your life!

6. **Eat Healthy.** If you want to feel good, look good and be happy, then eat healthy foods. Start your morning with a green smoothie or organic fruit juice. Eat a salad at lunch! Make sure that you're getting all of the essential nutrients your body needs to function properly. It's also important to understand that you need to drink plenty of clean water every day for you to be healthy, happy and whole. Make sure you're drinking at least eight 8-ounce glasses of clean, pure water daily to prevent dehydration and to keep your immune system strong.

7. **Help others.** We can never be truly happy until we help others, give back, and help make a difference in the lives of other people. If you want to be happy, then find ways to help people. Volunteer your time at a children's hospital, give to charities, help out at your local youth center or religious organization. Find any way you can to give, help, and share your gifts with the world. There are people in the world that need you to step up, guide them, teach them and show them the way. There are people close to you that need your

love, support and time. You can make a difference in the world, believe in your gifts, share your vision and give back!

8. **Be Honest.** Always be honest! Be honest with yourself, your family, friends, neighbors, boss, clients, wife, husband, everyone. Be honest! Honesty creates peace. Dishonesty creates chaos and misery. You don't need the added stress. Being dishonest in any way will cause you more pain than it's worth. If you want to be happy and live your life with joy, then be honest with everyone you come in contact with. There's no reason to lie about anything!

9. **No Complaining.** This is good. Complaining never works. It only magnifies and intensifies the thing that you're complaining about and makes it worse. Complaining never improves your situation: it's just a habit that needs to be broken if you truly want to be happy. It wasn't until I read *A Complaint Free World* by Will Bowen that I really started to pay attention to how much I actually complained. Check it out if you can. It's an amazing book and will help you take the initial steps to living a complaint-free life.

10. **Take Action.** The more action you take in the pursuit of your goals and dreams, the happier and luckier you will be. Activate your discipline and create the life you deserve. Without discipline, life will become unbearable. You need discipline to design the kind of life you have always dreamed of living. You need to take action, have a vision and see it through until the end. Taking massive amounts of action is the only way

for you to get from where you are to where you want to be. There's no other way. The more action you take, the happier you will be.

André Khabbazi

Smiling Works

Sometimes your joy is the source of your smile, but sometimes your smile can be the source of your joy.
— Thich Nhat Hanh

I grew up in a bad part of town. As a kid I was surrounded by gang members, drug dealers and tough kids who always for some reason wanted to tear my head off. I had to learn very quickly to give off a tough image, look mean and scowl, so I wouldn't get my face kicked in every day at school. Unfortunately, this habit stuck with me throughout my adult life.

It wasn't until a few years ago that I started to relax a bit and smile more at strangers. I let go of that tough image I had held on to for so many years, let my guard down and started smiling more just for the heck of it. Now, I smile all the time for no reason, even when I don't feel like smiling. It's impossible to be unhappy when you smile.

Try it for a day and see for yourself. Smile all day long. Smile at strangers, friends, family, your pet, your plants, your car, whatever. Just smile! Wipe that frown off your face for one day and replace it with a soft, beautiful smile. See how other people respond to you. Your stress will melt away; you will have more energy, look younger, be more approachable and stand out in the crowd.

Let go of the past. Today is a new day. Smile when you walk into a room even if you have to force it. If you see someone you dislike, smile at them and see how they respond to you. Smiling is contagious. Your smile will light up the world if you allow yourself to let go of your anxiety, fear and worries.

Your smile will make you more attractive, boost your immune system, encourage trust and send a signal to the universe that you're a happy human being. You will attract more amazing opportunities into your life, be more successful and find that inner harmony you've been searching for. Practice smiling. It's the best thing you can do to enhance the quality of your life. Smile! Smile! Smile!

André Khabbazi

Gratitude

Gratitude unlocks the fullness of life. It turns what we have into enough, and more. It turns denial into acceptance, chaos to order, confusion to clarity. It can turn a meal into a feast, a house into a home, a stranger into a friend.
— Melody Beattie

It's hard to be grateful for the little things when your life is a mess and you feel stuck. I spent 14 years working at a job that I hated, drinking, smoking and abusing my body. I blamed everyone for the terrible circumstances that I found myself stuck in and complained to anyone that would listen to my miserable story. All that did was cause me more pain, more frustration and more of the same thing.

It wasn't until I started applying the principles that I have been sharing with you throughout this book that my life stated to change for the better. I started exercising, reading, writing down my goals, visualizing, creating affirmations, eating healthier foods, juicing, and dreaming.

When I changed my habits, my life changed, and I was grateful for getting a second chance at life, grateful for becoming the person that I knew I was destined to be. It felt like my life changed overnight. I would go on a run in the mountains every morning and tears would run down my cheeks. I was grateful to be alive.

I would look up over the mountains, up into the blue sky and just say "thank you" for no reason, and I meant it. I felt it. I was overwhelmed with a sense of gratitude for all living things and wanted to express how I felt in words.

That's when I got the idea for this book. It just came to me out of thin air one morning. Like a flash of lightning behind the clouds.

I can appreciate my life now, more than ever. The small things: a smile, the sound of a familiar voice, breath, my fingers, my eyes, my ears, a beautiful song, a walk in the woods, the mountains, a stream. It's clear. Life is precious. It's a gift to be able to wake up each morning and start over. Another day of life. Another breath. Another smile. Another chance to help someone.

I'm going to give you a few ideas to play with that will hopefully inspire you and help you stay focused on all of the positive, amazing and wonderful things in your life!

3 Fun Ways to Cultivate Gratitude

The attitude of gratitude is closely related to that of contentment and is one of the greatest of all mental states; and the reason why is found in the fact that no mind can be right nor think constructively unless it is filled with the spirit of gratitude.

— Christian D. Larson

Step 1: Create a Gratitude Journal

Creating a gratitude journal is so much fun! You don't need a computer or a fancy notebook to get started. All you need is something to write with and a piece of paper and you're on your way. Find a quiet place to sit, where you can be alone and make a list of all the things you're grateful for in your life. Here are a few ideas to get you started:

- Your great health
- Your family
- Friends
- Love
- Your pets
- The weather
- A rainbow
- Nature
- Art

- A smile
- Meetings with strangers
- Laughter
- Books
- Generosity
- Change
- Fun
- Honesty
- Passion

As you can see there are no limits to what you can be grateful for. Creating a gratitude journal is a beautiful way to stop for a moment, slow down, breathe and realize that life is filled with a thousand little blessings that are often overlooked.

I enjoy writing in my gratitude journal first thing in the morning. This is a perfect time to make sure that I get it done, and it also sets the tone for my entire day. I can move through my day with a smile on my face, exuding love and gratitude to everyone that I come in contact with!

Step 2: Make a Habit of Always Saying "Thank You"

My world changed the moment I started repeating "thank you" for everything in my life. It opened my eyes to how magical life truly was. I stopped focusing on everything that was wrong and started to see the little miracles that life presented me in every moment.

You can do the same! I want to remind you as you go about your daily activities that your life is a blessing. The fact that you woke up today and you were given another chance at life is a true miracle. Look at yourself in the mirror before you leave the house today, look into your eyes and take notice of your breath. You're alive!

You've been given another chance to make this the best day of your life. Don't squander it, worrying yourself into the pits. Smile, remind yourself of all the blessings in your life and say "thank you" for everything that life puts in your path.

Step 3: The Blessings of Giving Back

There's no better feeling in the world than giving back and helping others. I believe that we were all put on this earth for the sole purpose of helping other human beings. We were put on this earth to be of service. To give, love, share, inspire and help people.

How do you feel when you help someone in need? My guess is that you feel amazing! It always feels good to be of service in some way. It takes the focus off of "you" and puts it on the person you're helping. The world is filled with people that need you. They need your smile, your love, your expertise, your financial support, your hard work, your words, and your talent. The world needs you!

So what can you do today, to put this into practice? I've written down a few simple ideas that will hopefully stimulate your imagination, motivate you to take action and start helping people:

- Random acts of kindness
- Acknowledge people; say "thank you"
- Smile at everyone
- Find ways to volunteer your time to help people in need
- Help family and friends
- Teach people a specific skill that you have
- Help out in your community
- Donate clothing to children
- Adopt a family during the holiday

We all live busy lives, but finding a few hours on the weekends or during the holidays to help people and give back will have a tremendous effect on the quality of your life. It only takes a moment to give someone a hug, a handshake, a kiss or a smile. It doesn't take much time to help your spouse do the dishes, clean the table or take out the trash.

You have so many wonderful things to be grateful for in your life. You have so much inside of you to give. Like I've said so many times before, the world needs you! Get out of your shell, spread your love and find a way to be of service to those who need you most.

Final Thoughts on Happiness

Try to make at least one person happy every day. If you cannot do a kind deed, speak a kind word. If you cannot speak a kind word, think a kind thought. Count up, if you can, the treasure of happiness that you would dispense in a week, in a year, in a lifetime!

— Lawrence G. Lovasik

Happiness is a choice. Smile at everyone you meet. Send love out to strangers, hug your children, your wife, your mother and your father. Tell the people you care about how much you love them. You will wake up one morning and they will be gone. Always tell the people that you care about how special they are to you. Never withhold your love. Give it. Send it out and share it with the world.

Cultivate gratitude for everything in your life. Every morning that you wake up and get out of bed is a day to celebrate. You made it. Go out and help someone in need. You were put on this earth to be of service. Give! Give! Give!

Choose your associations wisely. Surround yourself with people who are happy, positive and uplift your spirit. Stay away from complainers, whiners and negative people who suck your energy. There's only so much you can do to help those people. Most people don't want to change. They're stuck in the past and feel comfortable living in their own misery. If you let them, they will suck all of the positivity out of your life before you can even blink. Associate with people who inspire you, motivate you, and build you up.

Like I've said so many times throughout this book, you deserve to be happy, successful, healthy and abundant in every way. You were born into this world for a reason. Find that reason. Find your purpose. Don't get stagnant, comfortable or complacent. Don't ever get satisfied with where you are. Keep moving, keep searching, keep believing, and keep dreaming! Best of luck!

Conclusion

When you get into a tight place and everything goes against you, till it seems as though you could not hang on, hang on a minute longer, never give up then, for that is just the place and time that the tide will turn.

— Harriet Beecher Stowe

Congratulations! You made it through. You finished it. Give yourself a big hug for me. You're awesome! Thank you so much for going on this journey with me, and I sincerely hope that this book has a positive impact on the quality of your life. I'm so grateful for having the chance to share my ideas with you, inspire you, motivate you and hopefully guide you on your journey towards greatness!

My ultimate dream is to see you succeed in every area of your life and to live each day with love in your heart. You deserve that. You deserve to have it all! Affirm that every day and never forget how powerful, special and amazing you truly are. Find your purpose. Help people. Find a way to share your magic with the world and don't stop until you have accomplished all that you have set out to do.

It's up to you now to make that happen. I've given you a few tools to help you on your journey, but I need you to be strong, disciplined and willing to step out of your comfort zone. You can do it! Remember, life rewards action. Take action! Take one small step in the direction of your dreams and stay consistent with it. Consistency will be the key to your success, and your discipline will be the foundation for your greatness.

The more action you take, the luckier you will be. Keep that image of your dream close to your heart and never let it go. See it every morning when you wake up and hold on to it, no matter what obstacles come your way. You can do it!

My heart is with you!

Appendix

Green Smoothie and Juice Recipes for Superbeings

I will list some of my favorite juice and green super-smoothies for you. These are good to have anytime during the day when you need a little energy or just want to feel healthy and amazing! Enjoy!

NOTE: I use coconut water, alkaline water, or almond milk for the base in most of my green smoothies. I never use whole milk and rarely use soy milk. In my opinion, coconut water is the best!

I've left room for your personal notes on each recipe.

CITRUS BLAST — This juice combo is incredible! It's loaded with vitamin C and it tastes absolutely amazing.

- 3 oranges
- 2 grapefruits
- 1 lemon

Run it through your juicer and you're all set. This juice is refreshing, healing and will make your whole body tingle with joy. One of my favorite juice recipes.

WATERMELON BLISS — I love making this smoothie, especially in the morning or on a hot summer evening. Here's the basic recipe that I follow when making my Watermelon Bliss power smoothie.

- 1/2 of a watermelon
- 2 bananas
- 2 cups of coconut water (optional)
- pinch of bee pollen

Run it through your blender and you're all set to go. Yummy!

SUPER HERB MIRACLE SMOOTHIE — This smoothie will give you enough energy to last all day. It's loaded with superfoods, vitamins, and minerals. Great to drink before you exercise!

- 2 bananas
- dates
- cacao
- cacao nibs
- shou wu
- goji berries
- chia seeds
- flax seeds
- coconut water
- maca
- teaspoon of almond butter

I would usually start my day off with this mega-smoothie and have boundless energy the rest of my day. It's packed with some of the healthiest superfoods on the planet.

SUPERBEING PROTEIN JUICE — This packs a punch! This is one of my favorite, simple juice recipes. It gives you a ton of energy and makes you feel amazing.

- bunch of kale
- 2 stalks celery
- pinch of chlorella powder
- pinch of spirulina powder

GREEN SUPREME — This is a very refreshing green juice, it will help alkalize your body and send you off to work feeling like a superstar!

- bunch of kale
- 1 stalk celery
- 1 cucumber
- mint or parsley

COLD BUSTER — This recipe will help keep you healthy during the cold and flu season.

- a clove of garlic
- squeeze of fresh lemon
- an inch of ginger
- add honey
- add water
- add ice
- turmeric (optional)

Throw all ingredients into the blender, add some ice and mix.

DAILY GREEN JUICE — This is an incredible recipe I learned during my time at the Raw Food Institute. I suggest you drink this every morning if you can. It will keep you healthy, strong and energized all day long.

- 2 cucumbers
- 1/2 stalk celery
- 1/2 bunch parsley
- 1 lemon
- 1 clove garlic

Put all of the ingredients into your juicer, drink, and enjoy!

THE RED DEVIL — I love beets! Beets are loaded with antioxidants and are absolutely incredible for your health. When I get a sugar craving, this juice is high up there on my list. This is also my go to drink when I am feeling sick or tired. The ginger will spice things up and burn the cold or flu right out of your system.

- 1/2 beet
- 2 carrots
- 1 stalk celery
- 1/2 inch ginger

Put all ingredients into your juicer!

ABSOLUTELY PEAR — Pears are great to juice! If you are having a hard time drinking green juice, just add a pear. This drink is absolutely perfect.

- pear
- celery
- cucumber
- spinach

THE MEGA SUPER-SMOOTHIE — This smoothie is king!

- 3 cups coconut water
- cocoa
- 1 banana
- maca
- goji berries
- chai seeds
- flax seeds
- shilajit
- moringa leaf
- reishi
- chaga
- turmeric

Superfood Herbal Teas

Here are some of my favorite coffee alternatives that I've used over the years that taste amazing and are wonderful for your health.

GOLDEN MILK

- heat up 1 cup of water
- add 1/2 tsp. of turmeric
- small pinch of black pepper (pepper helps blood absorb the turmeric)
- add milk [Note: (I prefer almond milk or soy milk]
- let it simmer (do not boil)
- pour into a cup
- add honey and voila! Your Golden Milk is ready to drink.

SUPERFOOD LATTE — This is my favorite coffee alternative!

- warm water
- cacao powder
- maca powder
- chaga powder
- reishi powder
- cinnamon
- coffee optional

Blend all the ingredients together, and you will have your very own superfood latte.

Books That Will Change Your Life

I've listed here a few of my favorite books that have had the most impact on my life. Reading has been a big part of my world for the past 20 years and I am always searching for the next book that will take my life to the next level. I hope you get a chance to check out some of these amazing books and find the time to read a little bit every day. Good luck!

- *The Five Major Pieces to the Life Puzzle* (Jim Rohn)
- *Leading an Inspired Life* (Jim Rohn)
- *The Miracle Morning* (Hal Elrod)
- *The Sunfood Diet Success System* (David Wolfe)
- *Superfoods* (David Wolfe)
- *Chaga* (David Wolfe)
- *Longevity Now* (David Wolfe)
- *Think And Grow Rich* (Napoleon Hill)
- *The Slight Edge* (Jeff Olson)
- *The Power of Positive Thinking* (Norman Vincent Peale)
- *The 10x Rule* (Grant Cardone)
- *The War of Art* (Steven Pressfield)
- *The Science of Getting Rich* (Wallace D. Wattles)
- *Choose Yourself* (James Altucher)
- *The Magic of Thinking Big* (David J. Schwartz)
- *Make It Big* (Frank McKinney)
- *Ask and It Is Given* (Esther and Jerry Hicks)
- *Thinking for Results* (Christian D. Larson)

Books have the power to transform your life. Start reading, studying the masters and find mentors that will

help take your life to the next level.
Best of luck in all that you do,
André Khabbazi

About the Author

André Khabbazi is a successful American actor, writer and Brazilian jiu-jitsu enthusiast. He has starred in numerous TV shows including the lead role in the hit daytime drama The Young and the Restless and American Heiress. He has guest starred on hit shows 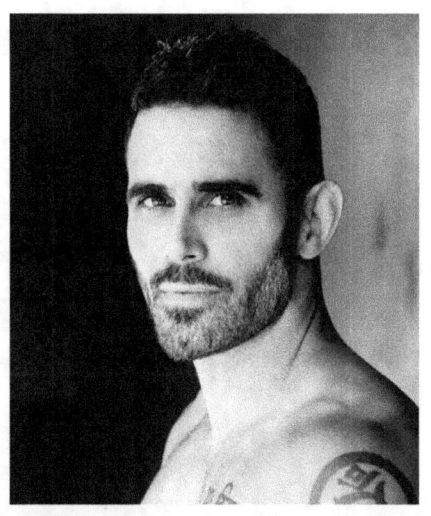 like CSI: Miami and CSI: New York, sharing the screen with Emmy award winning actor Gary Sinise. He is the co-author of a feature length screenplay, an acting coach, and spiritual adviser to artists in every medium around the globe.

For 20 years he has studied Homeopathic medicine,

Ayurvedic medicine, Kundalini yoga, Buddhist meditation and is a graduate of the The Raw Food Institute. In his spare time he enjoys spending time with his 3 beautiful children, reading, painting, and teaching Brazilian jiu-jitsu at the world renowned Charles Gracie Academy.

His love and passion for the arts have inspired him to create *The Superbeing Protocol,* and it is his mission to uplift thousands of people all over the world to get super fit, super healthy and to live their dreams. He firmly believes that anyone can change their life for the better if they take small consistent steps towards the realization of their goals, and never stop dreaming.